NATURAL TREATMENTS & REMEDIES

For The Worlds 400 Most Common Ailments

Global Health Research Institute

A GLOBAL HEALTH PUBLICATION

THIS PUBLICATION CONTAINS
REFERENCE INFORMATION ONLY
IT IS IN <u>NO WAY</u> INTENDED TO BE PRESCRIPTIVE OR DIAGNOSTIC.

This book is a reference work based on extensive research. The intent is to offer natural alternatives for complex solutions to treat the breakdown of the immunity system. In the event you use this information without your doctor's approval, you are prescribing for yourself, which is your constitutional right, but the publisher and author assume no responsibility.

Genesis 1: 29-30

"And God said, behold, I have given you every herb bearing seed, which is upon the face of all the earth, and every tree, in the which is the fruit of a tree yielding seed; to you it shall be for meat."

"And to every beast of the earth, and to every fowl of the air, and to everything that creepeth upon the earth, wherein there is life, I have given every green herb for meat: and it was so."

Global Health Ltd.
Box 18, Site 1, RR2
Tofield, Alberta, Canada
T0B 4J0

Canadian Cataloging in Publication Data
Nyholt, David H.
Natural treatments & remedies for the worlds 400 most common ailments.
Includes Bibliographical References and Index
1. Vitamin therapy. 2. Minerals in pharmacology. 3. Herbs - Therapeutic use. 4. Diet therapy. I Global Health Research. II Global Health Ltd. III. Title
RM259.N93 1994   615'.328   C94-910600-3
ISBN 0-921202-11-3

Printed in United States of America

DEDICATION

This book is dedicated to the multitudes who suffer needlessly; to the unprejudiced and dedicated healers that search out the natural remedies and treatments, to maintain and restore health without the risks of harmful side effects of synthetic drugs, and teach the principals with which to live a healthier life.

ACKNOWLEDGMENTS

We wish to express our sincere thanks to Global Health's research staff for their time, energy, and dedication. To David Nyholt for his wisdom and support in the preparation of this book, and to Shane Weatherill for the cover artwork.

FOREWORD

This book was assembled to provide the general public with the latest breakthroughs in natural health science and to keep you in touch with the proper natural treatments and remedies for the world's most common ailments. Nutrition should be looked upon as a means of preventing as well as treating disease. This can be accomplished through appropriate supplementation, proper selection of foods, and lifestyle changes. This guide will expand your awareness of treating yourself as naturally as possible, and discover a comfortable relationship with the latest natural alternatives for your busy lifestyle.

"Natural Treatments & Remedies" is one of the most comprehensive, concise, and straight forward natural health guide's on the market today. Simplified, allowing you to skim through and find what you want and need to know when you're at your busiest, or digest at your leisure. Using the quick scan index, clearly designed charts on vitamins, minerals, and R.D.A.'s give you more information in less reading time.

We are united in cause, to help you restore health, prevent premature aging, and prolong life for the continuing happiness and health of people around the world.

The Global Health Research Foundation.

CONTENTS

NATURAL TREATMENTS FOR 400 OF THE WORLD'S MOST COMMON AILMENTS

ABSCESS

SPECIFICS: An abscess forms when pus accumulates externally or internally in a particular part of the body due to infection. Most abscesses are treated with antibiotics which destroy the B vitamins as well as the friendly bacteria.

(Beneficial Remedies, Treatments, and Nutrients)

Single herbs: Burdock root, Cayenne, Chaparral, Dandelion root, Echinacea, Red Clover, Yellow Dock root.

Vitamins: A, B complex, E, C, plus a Multivitamin.

Minerals: Zinc, plus Mineral complex.

Also: Acidophilus, Garlic capsules, Pau d'arco, Raw Thymus, and Proteolytic enzymes.

Helpful foods: Beef, broccoli, carrots, fish liver oils, fruits, green leafy vegetables, herring, nuts, soybeans, spinach, pumpkin seeds, and whole wheat.

ACNE

SPECIFICS: A disorder of the oil(sebaceous) glands in the skin. It is believed that stress is a significant factor in acne. Other factors that contribute to acne are allergies, heredity, oral contraceptives, overindulgence in carbohydrates, and foods with high fat or sugar content and androgens(male hormones) produced in increased amounts when the girl or boy reaches puberty.

(Beneficial Remedies, Treatments, and Nutrients)

HERBAL COMBINATION: (AKN).

PHYSIOLOGIC ACTION: Acne is nearly always the product of blood impurities. AKN helps cleanse toxins and mucus. Enhances overall good health and well-being, and helps eliminate skin blemishes and acne.

Single herbs: Burdock, Chaparral, Chlorophyll, Echinacea, Garlic, Gotu Kola, Red Clover, Yellow Dock, and Yucca.

Vitamins: A, B complex, B3, B6, C, E, and F.

Minerals: Potassium, Sulfur, and Zinc.

Also: Primadophilus

Helpful foods: Avocados, bananas, broccoli, lean beef, carrots, celery, fruits (citrus and other), green leafy vegetables, pumpkin, radish, and vegetable oils.

ADRENAL EXHAUSTION

SPECIFICS: The adrenal glands are organs resting on top of each kidney. They are responsible for the production of the hormone epinephrine that speeds up the rate of metabolism in order to cope with stress and are involved in the metabolism of carbohydrates and the regulation of blood sugar. Adrenal exhaustion is most often caused by the long term use of cortisone drugs. Other causes are continuous stress, smoking, poor nutritional habits, and alcohol and drug abuse.

(Beneficial Remedies, Treatments, and Nutrients)

Single herbs: Astragalus, Echinacea, Milk Thistle, and Siberian Ginseng.

Vitamins: B2, B12, B complex, Folic acid, Pantothenic acid, C, and E.

Minerals: Copper, Potassium, Sodium, and Zinc.

Also: Coenzyme Q10, Germanium, L-Tyrosine, and Unsaturated fatty acids.

Helpful foods: Beef, broccoli, bananas, bacon, all fruits, herring, sea salt, raisins, soybeans, sweet potatoes, spinach, turnip greens, and whole wheat.

AGE SPOTS
(refer to Skin Problems - page 149)

AIDS
(Acquired Immune Deficiency Syndrome)
SPECIFICS: The virus that causes AIDS is called HIV, which stands for human immune deficiency virus. The virus is spread primarily through sexual contact or through the sharing of needles during intravenous drug use.

Building up the immune system is the best defense for the potential AIDS victim. The following nutrients can help the AIDS victim and those at risk to contact AIDS.

(Beneficial Remedies, Treatments, and Nutrients)

Single herbs: Cayenne, Chinese Ginseng, Garlic, Milk Thistle Weed, Shiitake mushroom, Sheep Sorrel, Suma, and Yucca.

Vitamins: A, B6, B12, B complex, and E.

Minerals: High potency multi-mineral formula, Copper, and Zinc.

Also: Canaid herbal drink, Acidophilus, Coenzyme Q10, Germanium, Gluconic from DaVinci Labs, Proteolytic enzymes, Quercetin plus bromelin, Raw thymus, and Multiglandulars.

AIR SICKNESS

SPECIFICS: Air sickness can indicate the presence of many diseases including inner ear infection, low blood sugar, food poisoning, and nutrient deficiency. The most common cause is a deficiency of the vitamin "B6", and the mineral "magnesium". Ginkgo is excellent for chronic dizziness and light headedness.

(Beneficial Remedies, Treatments, and Nutrients)

HERBAL COMBINATION: (Motion Mate).

PHYSIOLOGIC ACTION: In a recent university study ginger root caps proved more effective than either a drug or placebo at controlling motion induced nausea, also queasy travelers have found taking B complex at night and just before the trip is most effective.

Single herbs: Ginger Root Caps, and Ginkgo.

Vitamins: B complex plus B6.

Minerals: Magnesium.

Helpful foods: Fruits, lean beef, nuts, unpolished rice, whole grains, and yellow corn.

ALCOHOLISM

SPECIFICS: A chronic physiological or psychological condition marked by a dependence on alcohol. Deficiencies of many nutrients occur when alcohol itself satisfies the body's caloric needs. Some effects of alcohol are a depressed immune system, damage to the central nervous system, brain, duodenum, pancreas, liver, and a loss of inhibition.

Note: Tobacco, alcohol, caffeine and other drug "cravings" are brought about by a physiological body dependence on the poison which develops during prolonged use. The addicts blood poison level must remain at a certain level at all times. As the poison level drops, there is a "desire" to take in more of the drug, to bring the level back again.

(Beneficial Remedies, Treatments, and Nutrients)

HERBAL COMBINATIONS: (Thisilyn) (Milk Thistle) (PC) (Liveron) (AdrenAid).

PHYSIOLOGIC ACTION: The above herbal formulas support and rebuild the liver, pancreas, and adrenal glands. By supporting these systems, the taste for alcohol will eventually subside. The vitamin and mineral supplements strengthen the body's nutritional integrity to a state where the need for a "lift" will be eliminated.

Single herbs: Cayenne, Dandelion, Siberian Ginseng, Golden Seal, Licorice Root, Lobelia, Nettle, Skullcap, and Valerian.

Vitamins: A, B complex, B1, B2, B6, B12, Choline, Folic acid, Niacin, Pangamic acid, Pantothenic acid, C, D, E, and K.

Minerals: Calcium, Chromium, Iron, Magnesium, Manganese, Selenium, and Zinc.

Also: Acidophilus, Brewers Yeast, Glutamine, Liver, L-Cysteine, L-Glutamine, L-Methionine, Proteolytic enzymes, Tryptophan, Unsaturated fatty acids, and avoid meat and all refined and processed foods, especially white sugar and white flour.

Helpful foods: Butter, bran, broccoli, carrots, cheese, all fruits, green leafy vegetables, milk, peas, shellfish, spinach, and whole grains.

ALLERGIC RHINITIS
(refer to Hay Fever - page 80)

ALLERGIES

SPECIFICS: The inappropriate response by the body's immune system to some particular substance known as an allergen. The immune system wrongly identifies a non toxic allergen causing the white blood cells to overreact creating more damage to the body than the allergen itself.

The allergic reaction may cause asthma, dizziness, eczema, fever, hay fever, high blood pressure, hives, hypoglycemia, mental disorders, and stomach ulcers.

(Beneficial Remedies, Treatments, and Nutrients)

HERBAL COMBINATION: (HAS: Original and Fast Acting Formulas) (Allergy Care).

PHYSIOLOGIC ACTION: HAS is an excellent formula which contains herbs that help relieve symptoms of hay fever, sinus congestion, and respiratory allergies. Helps drain nasal passages, relieve swollen membranes, eliminate mucus, and cleanse the body. The Fast Acting Formula adds Pseudoephedra, a natural plant extract from the Ephedra plant. This substance quickly opens nasal passages allowing free breathing. While HAS Fast Acting is not for prolonged use, HAS Original can be taken for as long as needed.

WARNING: Both formulas are not to be used during pregnancy, nor by small children.

Allergy Care: Maximum-strength natural allergy medicine that will not cause drowsiness. It contains 60mg of the active ingredient Pseudoephedrine Hcl.

Single herbs: Burdock Root, Cayenne, Chaparral, Elderberry, Eyebright, Lobelia, Golden Rod, Golden Seal, and Nettles

HOMEOPATHIC COMBINATION: Allergy Formula

Vitamins: A, B complex, B3, B5, B6, B12, C, E, and F.

Minerals: A multi-mineral complex plus Calcium, Magnesium, Manganese, and Potassium.

Also: Acidophilus, Bee Pollen, Coenzyme Q10, Germanium, L-Tyrosine, L-Cysteine, Digestive Enzymes, Propolis, Raw adrenal, Raw thymus, and Unsaturated fatty acids.

Helpful foods: Almonds, apples, beef, beets, broccoli, carrots, cheese, bananas, fruits, safflower and linseed oil, spinach, and sweet potatoes.

ALOPECIA
(refer to Baldness - page 20)

ALZHEIMER'S DISEASE

SPECIFICS: Alzheimer's disease affects fifteen percent of Americans over the age of sixty five. This disease is characterized by tangled nerve fibers surrounding the brains memory center(hippocampus).

This entanglement does not destroy the information stored, but it can no longer be transferred to and from the brain. Science does not yet know what can be done to stop the mental deterioration, however autopsies of the victims of Alzheimer's disease show excess amounts of aluminum, bromine, calcium, silicon, and sulfur in the brain, and a deficiency of boron, potassium, selenium, zinc, and B12. in the brain. The excesses and deficiencies could be the key to the prevention or cure of Alzheimer's disease.

(Beneficial Remedies, Treatments, and Nutrients)

Single herbs: Butcher's Broom, Kelp, and Ginkgo Biloba.

Vitamins: B complex, plus B6, B12, C, and E.

Minerals: Boron, Potassium, Selenium, Vanadium, and Zinc.

Also: Coenzyme Q10, consume steam distilled water only, Germanium, Lecithin, Protein, and Superoxide dismutase.

Helpful foods: Beef, broccoli, bananas, bran, fish, green leafy vegetables, raisins, sweet potatoes, turnip greens, whole wheat, and all fruits.

ANCYLOSTOMIASIS

(refer to Hookworms - page 86)

ANEMIA

(Iron deficiency anemia)

SPECIFICS: The component of the blood that carries oxygen is hemoglobin, Iron is an important factor because this mineral makes hemoglobin, and the formation of red blood cells will be impaired by the lack of iron. Causes of iron deficiency anemia include heavy menstrual bleeding, hormonal disorders, liver damage, peptic ulcers, dierticular disease, thyroid disorders, and dietary disorders.

(Beneficial Remedies, Treatments, and Nutrients)

Single herbs: Barley Grass, Beet Powder, Black Current, Chlorophyll, Chorella, Comfrey, Dandelion, Fenugreek, Kelp, and Yellowdock.

Vitamins: A complete multi-vitamin and additional C.

Minerals: Complete multi-mineral.

Helpful foods: Broccoli, citrus fruits, sweet potatoes, turnip greens, red meat, whole rye, and black molasses.

Juices: Parsley and blackberry juice; parsley and grape juice.

ANGINA
(refer to Myocardial Infraction - page 117)

ANKYLOSING SPONDYLITIS

SPECIFICS: This condition is caused by inflammation affecting the joints between the vertebrae of the spine and the sacroiliac joints (the joints between the spine and the pelvis). Symptoms include stiffness and pain in the lower back, chest, and hips.

(Beneficial Remedies, Treatments, and Nutrients)

Single herbs: Devils Claw, Tumeric, and White Willow.

Vitamins: B6, B12, C, and E.

Minerals: Calcium and Magnesium.

Also: Bioflavonoids, Omega-3, Omega-6, Bromelain, and Digestive Enzymes.

Helpful foods: Broccoli, citrus fruits, kale, all green leafy vegetables, and whole grains.

ANOREXIA NERVOSA

SPECIFICS: In this disorder the individuals have an intense fear of becoming obese, and refuse to eat to the point of starvation. Symptoms include taking large doses of laxatives, deliberate vomiting, and self starvation. Recent studies show that some cases of anorexia nervosa may be caused by a severe zinc deficiency. When trying to stimulate the anorexic, consider the aroma and appearance of foods, as well as the nutritional value.

(Beneficial Remedies, Treatments, and Nutrients)

Single herbs: Catnip, Fennel, Ginger, Ginseng, Gotu Kola, Kelp, Papaya, Peppermint, and Saw Palmetto.

Vitamins: Multi-vitamins plus A, B12, B complex, D, and E.

Minerals: Multi-minerals plus Potassium, Selenium, and Zinc.

Also: Acidophilus, Bio-Strath, Brewer's yeast, Liver, Protein, and Proteolytic enzymes.

Helpful foods: Butter, bran, beef, bananas, herring, sunflower seeds, soybeans, spinach, tuna, and nuts.

ANURIA
(refer to Prostate and Kidney Disorders- page 136)

ANXIETY

SPECIFICS: Anxiety disorders affect roughly 4 percent of the population, mainly young adults. These disorders are generally a direct result of stress. The body can handle some stress but long term stress causes the body to break down. Long term stress occurs when the situation that causes anxiety is not relieved. Find the cause and handle it constructively. People experiencing anxiety should maintain a well-balanced diet and replace the nutrients depleted during stress.

(Beneficial Remedies, Treatments, and Nutrients)

HERBAL COMBINATIONS: (Calm-aid) or (Ex stress comb).

PHYSIOLOGIC ACTION: A proven formula that is soothing, strengthening, and healing to the whole nervous system to relieve nervous tension and rebuild the nerve sheaths. Excellent aid for insomnia, chronic nervousness, and stress-related conditions.

Single herbs: Evening Primrose Oil, Hops, Mistletoe, Skullcap, Valerian, and Yucca.

Vitamins: B complex, B1, B2, B3, B5, B6, and C.

Minerals: Calcium, Iodine, Iron, Magnesium, Phosphorus, Potassium, Silicon, and Sodium.

Helpful foods: Dulse, flax seed, sea salt, fruit(citrus and other), bacon, beef, chicken, all dairy products, all vegetables, and whole rye.

Juices: Radish and prune juice.

APTHOUS ULCERS

SPECIFICS: An apthous ulcer is a contagious and painful mouth ulceration that can appear on the lips, gums, tongue, and on the inside cheeks. The sores have white centers and are surrounded by a red border. Canker sores may be caused from eating to many sweets, poor dental hygiene or stress. They are identified by a tingling sensation and a slight swelling of the mucous membrane.

(Beneficial Remedies, Treatments, and Nutrients)

Single herbs: Goldenseal, Pau d'Arco, and Burdock Root tea, Red Clover, or Red Raspberry tea is very helpful.

Vitamins: A, B5, B12, B complex, and large doses of C.

Minerals: Iron.

Also: Acidophilus and L-Lysine.

Note: Avoid chewing gum, sugar, processed or refined foods, coffee, and citrus fruits.

Helpful foods: Black molasses, carrots, lean red meat, fish, leafy green vegetables, turnips, onions, potatoes, vegetable oils, and unpolished rice.

ARTERIOSCLEROSIS
(Hardening of arteries)

SPECIFICS: Arteriosclerosis is the thickening and hardening of the walls of the arteries. This condition is due to the gradual build-up of calcium and fatty deposits on the inside of the artery walls. This buildup will slow or restrict the circulation of the blood causing high blood pressure. Symptoms of arteriosclerosis are cramping of muscles, chest pains and pressure, and hypertension. Causes for arteriosclerosis are poor diet, drug abuse, alcoholism, smoking, heredity, obesity, and stress.

(Beneficial Remedies, Treatments, and Nutrients)

HERBAL COMBINATION: (Garlicin HC).

PHYSIOLOGIC ACTION: A combination of herbs which supports the cardiovascular system. Helps to strengthen the heart, while building and cleansing the arteries and veins.

SPECIFICS: Recent animal studies suggest that vitamin C deficiency could be involved in the causation of arteriosclerosis. E.F.A.s (essential fatty acids) play a fundamental role in keeping cell membranes fluid and flexible.

Single herbs: Cayenne, Comfrey, Evening Primrose Oil, Fish Oil, Garlic, Golden Seal, and Rose Hips.

Vitamins: B complex, C, E, Niacin, Inositol, and choline.

Minerals: Calcium and magnesium.

Also: (E.F.A.s) — Fish oils and cold pressed vegetable oils.

Helpful foods: Apples, lean beef, broccoli, fruits(citrus and other),sprouted seeds, sunflower seeds, sweet potatoes, sardines, tuna, turnip greens, and yellow corn.

ARTHRITIS

SPECIFICS: The most common forms of arthritis are osteoasthritis, and rheumatoid arthritis.

Rheumatoid arthritis is inflammatory in nature and attacks and destroys the synovial membranes surrounding the lubricating fluid in the joints. This damaged tissue is replaced with scar tissue, causing the space between the joints to narrow and to fuse together.

Osteoarthritis is a degenerative joint disease involving the deterioration of the cartilage at the ends of the bones, causing the cartilage to become rough resulting in friction.

(Beneficial Remedies, Treatments, and Nutrients)

HERBAL COMBINATION: (Rheum-Aid) or (Yucca -AR).

PHYSIOLOGIC ACTION: Relieves symptoms associated with bursitis, calcification, gout, rheumatoid arthritis, rheumatism, and osteoarthritis. Helps the body reduce or eliminate swelling and inflammation in the joints and connective tissue and helps to relieve stiffness and pain.

Single herbs: Alfalfa, Black Cohosh, Burdock, Cayenne, Celery seed, Chaparral, Devil's Claw, Valerian root, and Yucca.

HOMEOPATHIC COMBINATION: Arthritis Pain Formula.

Vitamins: Niacin, B5, B6, B12, B complex, C, D, E, F, and P.

Minerals: A strong Multi-mineral complex, plus Calcium, and Magnesium.

Also: Cod liver oil, Yu-ccan herbal drink, Green Magma, Aqua life, Seatone, and Bromelain.

Helpful foods: Almonds, apricots, beef, butter, broccoli, buckwheat, all fruits, cheese, sardines, soybeans, spinach, safflower, goats milk, and mung beans.

Juices: Parsley and celery juice; cherry and pineapple juice.

ASCARIASIS
(refer to Worms - page 174)

ASTHMA

SPECIFICS: A chronic respiratory condition caused by spasms in the muscles surrounding the small airways in the lungs called bronchi. Typical symptoms of asthma are coughing, difficulty in breathing usually accompanied by a wheezing sound, and a feeling of suffocation. The main causes of asthma are air pollution, respiratory infections, disorders of the adrenal glands, specific allergies, and physical or emotional stress.

(Beneficial Remedies, Treatments, and Nutrients)

HERBAL COMBINATIONS: (B R E) or (Breathe-Aid) and (ANTS Liquid Extract).

PHYSIOLOGIC ACTION: BRE or Breath-Aid effectively relieve symptoms associated with asthma, chest congestion, and inflammation. Promotes free breathing, eliminates mucus, and cleanses the body. ANTS Liquid Extract helps to relax bronchial spasms. It helps to cut mucus, and is helpful for chronic coughs.

Single herbs: Lobelia, Comfrey, Chlorophyll, Fenugreek, Mullein, and Nettle

Vitamins: A, B complex, B2, B3, B5, B6, B12, C, E, F, and Paba.

Minerals: Manganese.

Also: Bee pollen, honey (which will aid in clearing mucus out of the lungs), garlic, juice fast, and a vegetarian diet.

Helpful foods: Almonds, beets, broccoli, carrots, celery, all fruits, green leafy vegetables, nuts, peas, soybeans, spinach, and whole wheat.

Juices: Celery and papaya juice; carrot, celery, and endive juice.

ATHLETES FOOT

SPECIFICS: A highly contagious yeast like fungal infection, that lives off dead skin cells, and calluses of the feet. Athlete's foot victims should eat a well-balanced diet, supplemented by megadoses of vitamins A, B, and C.

(Beneficial Remedies, Treatments, and Nutrients)

HERBAL COMBINATION: (Black Walnut extract).

PHYSIOLOGIC ACTION: High in organic iodine, this herb has proven effective against fungal infections such as ringworm and athlete's foot.

Single herbs: Pau d'Arco and Tea Tree oil.

Vitamins: A, B complex, and C.

Minerals: Zinc.

Also: Acidophilus, Caprinex (caprylic acid), Germanium, and Unsaturated fatty acids. Vitamin C powder (crystals) applied directly to affected area helps destroy fungus infestation. Keep dry and out of shoes until infection clears.

Helpful foods: Red meats, all fruits, green leafy vegetables, herring, nuts, whole grains, and unpolished rice.

ATHLETIC INJURIES

SPECIFICS: Using the muscles for prolonged periods without rest can create muscle strain. If an athlete stresses a muscle beyond its capability the ligament connecting the bone to the muscle may tear causing a sprain. A well-balanced diet that is high in protein and the following supplement program will help these injuries heal.

(Beneficial Remedies, Treatments, and Nutrients)

HERBAL COMBINATION: (B F + C)

PHYSIOLOGIC ACTION: A special formula to aid in healing processes for torn cartilage's, sprained limbs, and broken bones. (Multiple athletic injuries and associated swelling and inflammation).

Single herbs: White Oak Bark, Comfrey Root, Black Walnut Hulls, Lobelia, Scullcap and Yucca.

HOMEOPATHIC COMBINATION: Injury and Backache Formula.

Vitamins: B complex, B5, B6, B12, C, and E.

Minerals: A complete multi-mineral one a day, (time released).

Also: Bee pollen, Coenzyme Q10, Germanium, L-Arginine, L-Carnitine, L-Lysine, Green-Lipped Mussel, Liver, Protein, Proteolytic enzymes, Silica, and Unsaturated fatty acids.

Helpful foods: Beef, fruits, nuts, unpolished rice, soybeans, spinach, vegetable oils, liver, and whole wheat.

Juices: Aloe Vera juice.

ATOPIC DERMATITIS

SPECIFICS: A type of skin eruption characterized by tiny blisters that weep and crust. Chronic forms produce flaking, scaling, itching, and eventual thickening and color changes of the skin.

(Beneficial Remedies, Treatments, and Nutrients)

HERBAL COMBINATION: (AKN).

PHYSIOLOGIC ACTION: When toxins are not properly eliminated from the body, they may surface through the skin creating atopic dermatitis. This formula has been created to support liver and gall bladder function, to ensure toxins are filtered from the blood.

Single herbs: Aloe Vera, Chickweed, Evening Primrose Oil, Pau d'Arco, Red Clover, Thisilyn (Milk Thistle), and Yellow Dock.

Vitamins: A, B complex, C, D, Paba, Biotin, Choline, and Inositol.

Minerals: Magnesium, Sulfur Ointment, and Zinc ointment.

Helpful foods: Apples, apricots, cherries, citrus fruits, all sea foods, lean red meat, chicken, broccoli, carrots, celery, vegetable oils, and grain sprouts.

Juices: Carrot, Celery, and Lemon juice.

Note: This condition is aggravated by food allergens such as dairy and wheat. These foods should be avoided. Powders and pastes should not be applied during acute or weeping stages. After acute stage passes, ointments and salves may be applied. Herbal ointments which contain Chickweed and Calendula are particularly helpful.

AUTISM

SPECIFICS: An illness that involves personalities of children who do not react to their environment. Children with autism are withdrawn, do not learn to talk or have learning disabilities, and exhibit marked unresponsiveness to affection and love. Scientific studies have shown that the combination of vitamin B6, and magnesium produces good results in children and adults with autism.

(Beneficial Remedies, Treatments, and Nutrients)

HERBAL COMBINATION: (Wild Lettuce and Valerian Extract).

PHYSIOLOGIC ACTION: This excellent formula is a natural sedative. Promotes overall calming of the nerves and restores a sense of control and balance without causing drowsiness.

Also: Ginkgo or Ginkgold. Although this herb is often used to promote circulation, it also has a positive effect on the nervous system. Used in conjunction with the following single herbs and with a balanced, chemical free diet, good results can be expected.

Single herbs: Evening Primrose Oil, Ginkgo, Lobelia, Oat Extract, Skullcap, St. Johns Wort, Valerian and Wild Lettuce.

Vitamins: High potency B vitamins, B3, B5, B6, and C.

Note: Yeast free B vitamins may be required if yeast intolerance is present.

Minerals: High doses of all minerals.

Note: Avoid all foods with artificial flavoring and coloring. Processed foods should be eliminated from the diet. Foods which contain natural salicylates such as apples, tomatoes, and oranges need to be avoided. Carbonated drinks will worsen the condition.

Helpful foods: Beets, broccoli, fruits, nuts, sweet potatoes, turnip greens, peas, and unpolished rice.

AUTOIMMUNE DISORDERS

SPECIFICS: When the immune system weakens and is unable to respond to invading microorganisms you become more susceptible to infections and viruses. The key factors in the treatment and prevention of autoimmune disorders are proper nutrition and good supplementation.

(Beneficial Remedies, Treatments, and Nutrients)

HERBAL COMBINATION: (EchinaGuard).

PHYSIOLOGIC ACTION: Stimulates the immune response systems. Especially helpful in rebuilding the body during convalescence and as a preventative.

Single herbs: Echinacea root, Chaparral, Evening Primrose, Korean White Ginseng, Goldenseal root, Pau d'Arco, and Rosemary.

Vitamins: A multi-vitamin plus B6, B12, C, and E.

Minerals: A strong mineral complex.

Also: Canaid herbal drink, L-Cysteine, L-Methionine, L-Lysine, L-Ornithine, Omega-3, Omega-6, Propolis, Proteolytic enzymes, and Primadophilus.

Helpful foods: Beef, broccoli, fruit(citrus and other), nuts, soybeans, spinach, sweet potatoes, turnip greens, unpolished rice, and whole grains.

BACK PAIN

SPECIFICS: Most back problems are associated with long term habits. Chronic pain in the lower back is usually caused by improper footwear, sleeping on a mattress that is too soft, poor posture, and walking habits.

(Beneficial Remedies, Treatments, and Nutrients)

HERBAL COMBINATIONS: (Extress) (Kalmin Extract)

PHYSIOLOGIC ACTION: The herbs in these combinations help to relax muscles and reduce muscle tension. The Kalmin Extract has anti-spasmodic and anti-inflammatory qualities which are helpful in back pain caused by muscle strain.

Single herbs: Burdock, Horsetail, Licorice, Valerian, and White Willow Bark.

Vitamins: B12, C D, and E,

Minerals: Calcium, Magnesium, Manganese, Silicon, and Zinc.

Also: Cod liver oil, Enzymes with bromelin, DL-Phenylalanine, L-Tryptophan, and Protein.

Helpful foods: All dairy products, beef, cod liver oil, tuna, beets, broccoli, peanuts, sunflower seeds, soybeans, and sprouted seeds.

BAD BREATH

SPECIFICS: Bad breath is generally attributed to putrefactive bacteria living on undigested food. Nutrients necessary for efficient digestion are essential. Other causes are poor dental hygiene (gum or tooth decay), nose or throat infection, excessive smoking, liver malfunction, and constipation.

(Beneficial Remedies, Treatments, and Nutrients)

Single herbs: Chlorophyll, Myrrh, Parsley, Peppermint, Rosemary, Sage, and Yucca.

Vitamins: A, B complex, B3, B6, C, and Paba.

Minerals: Magnesium, and Zinc.

Also: Primadophilus, Digestive enzymes, and Yu-ccan herbal drink.

Helpful foods: Apples, carrots, citrus fruits, and parsley.

BALDNESS

SPECIFICS: There is no known cure to hair loss in males due to heredity. If one is a victim of hair loss due to acute illness, pregnancy, surgery, poor circulation, or stress, the following nutrients can be helpful.

(Beneficial Remedies, Treatments, and Nutrients)

Single herbs: Aloe Vera, Horsetail, Kelp, Rosemary, Sage, Nettle, Yarrow, and Yucca.

Vitamins: A, B complex, B3, B5, B6. C, Biotin, Folic Acid, and Inositol.

Minerals: Copper, Iodine, Magnesium.

Also: Coenzyme Q10, L-Cysteine, L-Methionine, Primadophilus, Protein, Raw thymus glandular, and Unsaturated fatty acids.

Helpful foods: Asparagus, broccoli, cabbage, beef, seafood, fish liver oils, all fruit, green leafy vegetables, turnip greens, and unpolished rice.

BEDSORES

SPECIFICS: Bedsores are deep skin ulcers that are the result of continuous pressure exerted over bony areas restricting circulation and leading to the death of skin tissue. Massaging the affected area daily is very helpful. Frequent sponge baths with warm water and a mild herbal soap or a soap containing vitamin E are recommended.

(Beneficial Remedies, Treatments, and Nutrients)

HERBAL COMBINATION: (X-Itch ointment)(Derm-Aid ointment)

PHYSIOLOGIC ACTION: X-Itch, and Derm-Aid are used for the relief and prevention of minor skin irritations. Black ointment has a drawing and healing effect for those tough to heal sores.

Single herbs: Goldenseal, Myrrh gum, and Pau d' Arco.

Vitamins: A, B complex, C, D, and E.

Minerals: Copper, Calcium, Magnesium, and Zinc.

Helpful foods: Beef, butter, cheese, all fruits, tuna, fish liver oils, nuts, and sunflower seeds.

BED-WETTING

SPECIFICS: The exact cause of bed-wetting(nocturnal enuresis) is still unknown, however it is believed that nervous or hyperactive children, and children having a faster heart beat and higher respiration rate during the sleep cycle are more likely to be bed-wetters. The most common theories speculate that the causes may be heredity, behavioral disturbances, stress, weak bladders, urinary tract infections, and nutritional deficiencies.

(Beneficial Remedies, Treatments, and Nutrients)

Single herbs: Buchu, Corn silk, Oat straw, Parsley, and Plantain.

Vitamins: A multi-vitamin plus A, B complex, and E.

Minerals: A mineral complex plus Potassium, and Zinc.

Also: Cod liver oil, and Protein.

Helpful foods: Celery and parsley juice.

BEE STINGS

SPECIFICS: If stung, a very severe reaction can occur to people that are allergic to bee venom. Symptoms include severe swelling, labored breathing, hoarseness, confusion, difficulty in swallowing, and weakness. If you have a known allergy to bee stings, have your doctor prescribe an emergency treatment kit.

(Beneficial Remedies, Treatments, and Nutrients)

Single herbs: Echinacea, Pau d'Arco, and Yellow Dock tea.

Vitamins: B1 is a good insect repellent, and it creates a smell at the level of the skin that insects do not like. Already stung, use vitamin C to ease allergic reaction (acts as a natural anti-histamine).

Minerals: Calcium.

Helpful foods: Citrus fruits, turnip greens, all dairy products, and sardines.

BELCHING
(refer to Gas "Intestinal" - page 71)

BERIBERI

SPECIFICS: A disease caused by a deficiency of B vitamins, particularly thiamine. The disease seldom occurs outside the Far East, where the principal diet of polished rice does not supply sufficient thiamine. Beriberi cases that do occur in America are associated with chronic alcoholism, hypothyroidism, infections, pregnancy, and stress.

(Beneficial Remedies, Treatments, and Nutrients)

Vitamins: B1, B complex, and C.

Minerals: A complete mineral complex.

Also: Brewers yeast.

Helpful foods: Beef, broccoli, fruits(citrus and other), nuts, sweet potatoes, and turnip greens,

BIPOLAR DISORDER

SPECIFICS: A mental disorder characterized by swings in mood between opposite extremes. Mood swings may be accompanied by extreme negative delusions or by grandiose ideas. The main causes of this ailment are drugs, inherited tendency, and malnutrition.

(Beneficial Remedies, Treatments, and Nutrients)

Vitamins: B complex, B12, and Folic Acid.

Minerals: Lithium.

Also: Omega-6 oils, L-phenylalanine, and L-tryptophan.

Helpful foods: Liver, red meat, eggs, asparagus, citrus fruits, turnip greens, sprouted seeds, cheese and other dairy products, sunflower seeds, wheat germ, and whole grains.

BLADDER INFECTION
(refer to Kidney and Bladder Disorders - page 96)

BLEEDING GUMS

SPECIFICS: Bleeding gums are nearly always caused by a nutrient deficiency. The recommended prevention and treatment is a well-balanced diet that is rich in all nutrients.

(Beneficial Remedies, Treatments, and Nutrients)

Single herbs: Chamomile, Echinacea, Lobelia, Myrrh Gum, and White Oak Bark.

Vitamins: A, B complex, C, D, P, and Folic Acid.

Minerals: Calcium, Magnesium, Phosphorus, and Silicon.

Helpful foods: Apple, apricots, corn, carrots, butter, cheese, tuna, fish liver oils, green leafy vegetables, peanuts, sunflower seeds, and sprouted seeds.

BLOOD CLEANSER

SPECIFICS: If you are run down and full of toxins, watch out! A person should cleanse his or her blood at least once every six months, to eliminate the germs that live on the mucus, toxins, and poisons in the body.

(Beneficial Remedies, Treatments, and Nutrients)

HERBAL COMBINATION: (Red Clover combination)

PHYSIOLOGIC ACTION: Helps cleanse the blood of toxins, mucus, and infections thus helps improve and sustain overall good health; used for many years with very good results.

Single herbs: Red Clover, Chaparral, Dandelion, Garlic, and Burdock.

Minerals: Iron.

Also: Chlorophyll and Diulaxa tea.

Helpful foods: Black molasses, carrots, celery, parsley, red meat, tomatoes, and whole rye.

Juices: Blackberry, blackcherry, carrot, celery, dandelion, parsley, and tomato juice.

BLOOD CLOTS

SPECIFICS: Blood clots are due to the gradual build-up of calcium and cholesterol-containing masses known as plaques on the inside of the artery walls. The clot will slow or restrict the circulation of the blood causing high blood pressure. Symptoms of this disease are cramping of muscles, chest pains and pressure, and hypertension. The main causes are poor diet, drug abuse, alcoholism, smoking, heredity, obesity, and stress.

(Beneficial Remedies, Treatments, and Nutrients)

HERBAL COMBINATION: (Garlicin HC).

PHYSIOLOGIC ACTION: A combination of herbs which supports the cardiovascular system. Helps to strengthen the heart, while building and cleansing the arteries and veins.

SPECIFICS: Recent animal studies suggest that vitamin C deficiency could be involved in the causation of thrombosis. E.F.A.s (essential fatty acids) play a fundamental role in keeping cell membranes fluid and flexible.

Single herbs: Cayenne, Comfrey, Evening Primrose Oil, Fish Oil, Garlic, Golden Seal, and Rose Hips.

Vitamins: B complex, C, E, Niacin, Inositol, and Choline.

Minerals: Calcium, Magnesium, and Selenium.

Also: (E.F.A.s) — Fish oils and cold pressed vegetable oils.

Helpful foods: Fish and fish liver oils, vegetable oils, oat bran, high fiber fruits, kelp, green tea, yogurt, and legumes.

Juices: Alfalfa, beet, blackberry, grape, parsley, and pineapple juice.

BLOOD PRESSURE *(High)*

SPECIFICS: The main cause of high blood pressure is arteriosclerosis. This condition is due to the gradual build-up of calcium and fatty deposits on the inside of the artery walls. This buildup will slow or restrict the circulation of the blood causing high blood pressure. Symptoms of high blood pressure are cramping of muscles, chest pains and pressure, and hypertension. Causes for high blood pressure are poor diet, drug abuse, alcoholism, smoking, heredity, obesity, and stress.

(Beneficial Remedies, Treatments, and Nutrients)

HERBAL COMBINATIONS: (Cayenne-Garlic) (Garlicin HC) (BP)

PHYSIOLOGIC ACTION: In addition to lowering the blood pressure, the above will help to relieve colds, influenza, and general infections, strengthen the heart and improves blood circulation.

Single herbs: Cayenne, Garlic, Kelp, Hawthorn, Mistletoe, Valerian Root, Yarrow, and Yucca.

Vitamins: A, B complex (stress) B3, B5, B15, C, D, E, P, Inositol, Choline, and Lecithin

Minerals: Calcium, Magnesium, and Potassium.

Helpful foods: Apples, apricots, bananas, cherries, broccoli, carrots, green leafy vegetables, soybeans, sunflower seeds, vegetable oils, and fish liver oils.

Juices: Carrot, celery, grape, and lime juice.

BLOOD PRESSURE (LOW)

SPECIFICS: There are many disorders associated with circulatory problems. The most common disease for sluggish circulation is Raynaud's disease, characterized by constriction and spasm of the blood vessels in the limbs. Poor circulation can also result from varicose veins, caused by the loss of elasticity in the walls of the veins.

(Beneficial Remedies, Treatments, and Nutrients)

HERBAL COMBINATION: (B/P).

PHYSIOLOGIC ACTION: A time proven formula that improves overall blood circulation and tends to normalize high or low pressure to the body's normal level. Also reduces cholesterol build-up in the blood vessels. Helps relieve symptoms of cold and flu.

Single herbs: Garlic, Hawthorn, Siberian Ginseng, Kelp, Golden Seal Root, Ginger Root, and Spirulina,

Vitamins: A, B Complex, B5, C, E, and P.

Also: EPA. Salmon oil, and Lecithin.

Helpful foods: Fruits(citrus and other), carrots, broccoli, spinach, lean beef, and all seafood's.

BODY ODOR

SPECIFICS: Most body odors are related to the internal health of the body, caused by sluggish or infected bowel, kidney, or bladder. Certain nutrients such as the B vitamins, magnesium, and zinc appear to remove wastes in the body that cause odors.

(Beneficial Remedies, Treatments, and Nutrients)

Vitamins: B6, PABA, and B complex.

Minerals: Magnesium, and Zinc.

Also: Chlorophyll and Yu-ccan herbal drink.

Helpful foods: Brewers yeast, nuts, fruits, unpolished rice, and whole grains.

BOILS

SPECIFICS: A painful localized infection producing pus filled areas in the deeper layers of the skin tissues. A boil forms when the skin tissue is weakened by chafing and there is inadequate nutrition to fight infection. Treatment for boils demands proper hygiene, frequent washing with soap and water, and application of an antiseptic.

(Beneficial Remedies, Treatments, and Nutrients)

HERBAL COMBINATION: (AKN).

PHYSIOLOGIC ACTION: Many skin diseases such as boils are often related to liver dysfunction. This herbal formula combines herbs which support the liver, and clean the blood.

FOR PAIN: Make a paste of wheat flour and honey, spread over area, and cover with cotton dressing.

Single herbs: Chaparral, Dandelion, Echinacea, Lobelia, Mullein, and Red Clover.

Vitamins: A, C, E. Vitamin A may be applied locally.

Minerals: Zinc (preventative).

Helpful foods: Citrus fruits, herring, tuna, fish liver oils, soybeans, sunflower seeds, carrots, sweet potatoes, turnip greens, and melon.

BONE, FLESH AND CARTILAGE

(Disorders)

SPECIFICS: Using the muscles for prolonged periods without rest can create muscle strain. If an athlete stresses a muscle beyond its capability the ligament connecting the bone to the muscle may tear causing a sprain. A well-balanced diet that is high in protein and the following supplement program will help these injuries heal.

(Beneficial Remedies, Treatments, and Nutrients)

HERBAL COMBINATION: (BF + C).

PHYSIOLOGIC ACTION: A special formula to aid the body's healing processes involved with broken bones, athletic injuries, sprained limbs, and related inflammation and swelling. A tonic used after acute and chronic diseases to help rebuild the body.

Single herbs: Comfrey Root, Black Walnut, Horsetail, Lobelia, Skullcap, White Oak Bark, and Yucca.

HOMEOPATHIC COMBINATION: Injury and Backache Formula.

Vitamins: A, Pantothenic acid, C, and D.

Minerals: Calcium, Magnesium, and Potassium.

Note: Protein and silicon accelerate bone healing.

Helpful foods: Beef, tuna, fish liver oils, all dairy products, citrus fruits, carrots, green and green leafy vegetables, nuts, seeds, and sprouted seeds.

BONE SPUR
(refer to Heel Spur - page 83)

BOWEL CLEANSER *(Lower)*

SPECIFICS: Constipation results when the waste material moves too slowly or there is decreased frequency of bowel movements. Constipation usually arises from insufficient amounts of fiber and fluids in the diet. Other causes include lack of exercise, nervousness, stress, infections, and poor diet.

(Beneficial Remedies, Treatments, and Nutrients)

HERBAL COMBINATION: (Multilax #2) or (Naturalax #2).

PHYSIOLOGIC ACTION: Accelerates natural cleansing of the body and improves intestinal absorption by gentle evacuation of the bowels. It cleans out old, toxic fecal matter, mucus and encrustation's from the colon wall, and helps normalize the peristaltic action and rebuild the bowel structure. Use until the bowel is cleansed, healed, and functioning normally.

WARNING: Do not take during pregnancy.

Single herbs: Cascara Sagrada, Golden Seal Root, Lobelia, Red Raspberry, Senna, and Yucca.

Vitamins: B complex.

Also: Yogurt, soaked Prunes and Figs, and Yu-ccan herbal drink.

Helpful foods: Brewers yeast, flax seed, fruits, lean beef, nuts, prunes, unpolished rice, whey powder, and yogurt.

BREAST CANCER
(refer to Cancer - page 34)

BREAST FEEDING

SPECIFICS: The three main breast feeding problems are:

- ENGORGEMENT; which results in the swelling of the tissues in the breast causing the breasts to feel full, hard, and tender. Treatment and prevention of this disorder includes short frequent feedings and the non restriction of sucking time.

- SORE NIPPLES; this is usually caused by improper nursing schedules and improper nursing positions.

- PLUGGED DUCT; this is usually caused by a tiny clot of dried milk plugging the nipple, or incomplete emptying of the milk ducts. If the breast is infected refer to <u>Mastitis</u> in this manual.

(Beneficial Remedies, Treatments, and Nutrients)

Single herbs: Alfalfa, Blessed Thistle, Chlorophyll, Fennel, Red Raspberry, or Marshmallow (warm) will bring in good rich milk. Sage will help dry up the milk when the mother is ready to quit nursing.

Vitamins: If the baby has a cold, the mother can take extra vitamin C.

WARNING: A nursing mother should not take cleansing herbs as it may cause colic or diarrhea in the baby.

BREATHING DIFFICULTIES

SPECIFICS: The main causes of breathing difficulties are air pollution, respiratory infections, disorders of the adrenal glands, specific allergies, and physical or emotional stress. Also refer to asthma, and bronchitis in this manual.

(Beneficial Remedies, Treatments, and Nutrients)

HERBAL COMBINATIONS: (B R E) or (Breathe-Aid) (Fenu-Comf)

PHYSIOLOGIC ACTION: Effectively relieves irritation and promotes healing throughout the respiratory tract. Eliminates mucus, inflammation of the lungs, and helps relieve symptoms of coughs, colds, and bronchitis.

Single herbs: Comfrey Leaves, Lobelia, Marshmallow Root, and Mullein.

Vitamins: C.

Also: Respa-Herb and Bee Pollen.

Helpful foods: Broccoli, citrus fruits, and turnip greens.

BRIGHTS DISEASE

SPECIFICS: A chronic inflammation of the kidneys, characterized by blood in the urine with associated hypertension and edema which results in the kidney retaining salt and water. When the bloodstream becomes toxic with wastes due to kidney malfunction, uremia develops. The following nutrients will aid in controlling urinary tract infection.

(Beneficial Remedies, Treatments, and Nutrients)

HERBAL COMBINATION: (KB).

PHYSIOLOGIC ACTION: Extremely valuable in healing and strengthening the kidneys, bladder, and genito-urinary area.

Useful to stop bed-wetting, but is a diuretic when congestion of the kidneys is indicated. Helps remove bladder, uterine, and urethral toxins.

WARNING: Intended for occasional use only. May cause green-yellow discoloration of the urine.

Vitamins: A, B complex, C, D, E, Choline.

Single herbs: Alfalfa, Barberry root, Catnip, Dandelion, Fennel, Ginger root, Horsetail, and Wild Yam.

Also: Cranberry juice, Propolis, Uratonic, 3-way herb teas, and other Diuretic tablets.

Helpful foods: Lean red meat, carrots, soybeans, tuna, fish liver oils, all fruits, and sprouted seeds.

BRONCHITIS

SPECIFICS: An inflammation of the tissues lining the air passage, or obstruction of the breathing tubes that lead to the lungs. The inflammation is usually followed by a mucus buildup, coughing, sore throat, fever, and back and chest pains. The main causes of bronchitis are air pollution, fatigue, malnutrition, and cigarette smoking. Treatment requires a well-balanced diet high in vitamins A and C.

(Beneficial Remedies, Treatments, and Nutrients)

HERBAL COMBINATION: (Fenu-Comf).

PHYSIOLOGIC ACTION: Helps relieve symptoms of coughs, colds, bronchitis, and helps eliminate mucus, congestion, and inflammation from the lungs.

Single herbs: Comfrey, Eucalyptus, Lobelia, Chickweed Tea, Slippery Elm. Cayenne taken with Ginger cleans out the bronchial tubes.

Vitamins: A, B12, C, and E.

Minerals: A multi-mineral formula plus Zinc.

Also: Acidophilus, Coenzyme Q10, L-Arginine, L-Cysteine, L-Ornithine, Protein, Proteolytic enzymes, and Unsaturated fatty acids.

Helpful foods: Citrus fruits, fish liver oils, carrots, sweet potatoes, and turnip greens.

Juices: Lemon juice with honey.

BRUISES

SPECIFICS: An injury that involves the rupture of small blood vessels resulting in swelling and black and blue marks due to the blood that has collected under the skin. The most common factors that make a person susceptible to bruises are anemia, time of menstrual period, and being overweight. The following nutrients can be helpful in the prevention and treatment of bruises.

(Beneficial Remedies, Treatments, and Nutrients)

Single herbs: Alfalfa, Garlic, and Rosehips.

Vitamins: B9, B complex, C, D, E, and K.

Minerals: Calcium, Iron, and Magnesium.

Also: Germanium, Proteolytic enzymes, and Coenzyme Q10.

Helpful foods: Beef, butter cheese, all fruits, kelp, liver, soybeans, sunflower seeds, spinach, sprouted seeds, whole wheat, and yogurt.

BRUXISM
(refer to Teeth Grinding - page 156)

BURNING FEET

SPECIFICS: Burning feet are caused by a deficiency of B6, B12, and Iron.

(Beneficial Remedies, Treatments, and Nutrients)

Vitamins: B6 and B12.

Minerals: Iron.

Helpful foods: Black molasses, citrus fruit, nuts, and whole rye.

BURNING MOUTH AND TONGUE

SPECIFICS: Nearly all mouth and tongue disorders such as sore mouth, tongue, and gums are attributed to a deficiency of the B vitamins. The gums become puffy, tender, and the oral membranes become susceptible to canker sores with the deficiency of vitamin C and niacin.

(Beneficial Remedies, Treatments, and Nutrients)

Single herbs: Aloe Vera, Golden Seal, Myrrh, Red Raspberry, and White Oak Bark.

Vitamins: A, B complex, B2, B3, B12, C, and E.

Minerals: Iron, Magnesium, Phosphorus, and Zinc.

Also: Chlorophyll, Lysine, and Primadophilus.

Helpful foods: All fruits, carrots, corn, broccoli, herring, oysters, red meat, soybeans, and spinach.

BURNS

SPECIFICS: There are three degrees of burns. The first degree burn appears reddened, the second degree burn appears reddened and includes blisters, in the third degree burn the entire thickness of the
skin is destroyed and possibly the underlying muscle. For third degree burns immediate treatment is required, see your doctor.

(Beneficial Remedies, Treatments, and Nutrients)

Single herbs: Aloe Vera, and Comfrey.

PHYSIOLOGIC ACTION: Aloe Vera is very good for burns, it may be used internally and externally. Some Aloe Vera preparations contain lanolin, which will intensify burns. Use a preparation without lanolin. Aloe Vera is especially good for acid burns.

Vitamins: A, C, E, Niacin, Paba. (Vit E applied directly to burn). Take vitamin C hourly-this will help prevent infection from occurring.

Minerals: Calcium, Magnesium, Potassium, and Zinc.

Also: Ice, cold water, Paba cream, liquid honey, Comfrey poultice.

Helpful foods: Apples, bananas, broccoli, carrots, cheese, citrus fruits, herring, fish liver oils, green leafy vegetables, turnip greens, and vegetable oils.

BURSITIS

SPECIFICS: Bursitis is an inflammation of the bursae, liquid filled sacs found in the joints, tendons, muscles, and bones. This disorder is commonly found in the elbow, hip, and shoulder joints, causing swelling, tenderness, and extreme pain. During infection, elevated doses of A, C, and E are beneficial in the treatment of bursitis.

(Beneficial Remedies, Treatments, and Nutrients)

HERBAL COMBINATIONS: (Rheum-Aid) (Cal-Silica) (Kalmin).

PHYSIOLOGIC ACTIONS: These herbal combinations contain herbs which exhibit anti-inflammatory and relaxing effects. Help to build nerve tissue and relieve stiffness and pain.

Single herbs: Alfalfa, Chaparral, Comfrey, and Yucca. Mullein is often used as a poultice to give relief externally.

Vitamins: A, B12, B complex, C, E, and P.

Minerals: Calcium and Magnesium.

Also: Alkaline diet, Coenzyme Q10, Germanium, Proteolytic enzymes, Yu-ccan herbal drink, and a protein supplement.

Helpful foods: Apples, apricots, cherries, citrus fruits, sardines, tuna, fish liver oils, spinach, and sweet potatoes.

CADMIUM TOXICITY

SPECIFICS: Cadmium is a tin like metal. Poisoning is usually due to breathing in cadmium dust and fumes by industrial workers. This problem may also arise when people consume foods that have been stored in cadmium lined containers. This metal has been linked to the development of high blood pressure and acute exposure can lead to kidney failure and permanent lung damage. Cadmium levels are much higher in smokers and non smokers may also accumulate higher levels from second hand smoke.

(Beneficial Remedies, Treatments, and Nutrients)

Single herbs: Alfalfa and Garlic.

Vitamins: E.

Minerals: Calcium, Copper, Magnesium, and Zinc.

Also: L-Cysteiene, L-Lysine, and L-Methionine.

Helpful foods: Whole grains, fibrous fruits, pumpkin seeds, and other foods that have a high zinc content.

CALAMYDIA

SPECIFICS: Calamydia is the most common sexually transmitted disease. The microorganisms that cause this disease, can also be passed from the mother to the newborn infant, as it passes through the infected birth canal. Complications of calamydia may result in sterility in both sexes. Penicillin or another antibiotic is the usual treatment. In addition to medical treatment, an afflicted person should maintain a high nutrient diet to help repair the tissue damage that has occurred.

(Beneficial Remedies, Treatments, and Nutrients)

Single herbs: Echinacea, Goldenseal, Kelp, Pau d'Arco, Red Clover, and Suma.

Vitamins: A, B complex, C, E, and K.

Minerals: Zinc.

Also: Acidophilus, Coenzyme Q10, Germanium, and Proteolytic Enzymes.

Helpful foods: All red meats, cabbage, fruits, aloe vera, kelp, herring, oysters, liver, nuts, and yogurt.

CALCIUM DEFICIENCY

SPECIFICS: Low levels of calcium in the blood may seriously disrupt cell function in muscles and nerves. Vitamin D will help control the overall amount of calcium in the body by regulating the amount of calcium removed from the body by the kidneys and the amount absorbed from food.

(Beneficial Remedies, Treatments, and Nutrients)

HERBAL COMBINATION: (Ca -T).

PHYSIOLOGIC ACTION: This proven formula contains organic calcium, silica, and other tranquilizing minerals help prevent cramps. A natural way to calm nerves and aid sleep in addition to rebuilding the nerve sheath, vein, artery walls, teeth, and bones.

Single herbs: Comfrey Root, Horsetail, and Lobelia.

Vitamins: D.

Minerals: Calcium.

Helpful foods: Dark green leafy vegetables such as kale, mustard greens, collard greens, cabbage, broccoli are rich sources of easily assimilated calcium. Foods such as lentils, almonds, and sesame seeds are other good sources.

CALCULUS
(refer to Kidney and Bladder Stones - page 97)

CANCER

SPECIFICS: With cancer, cells begin to reproduce for no obvious reason. The cancer cells rob the normal cells of their essential nutrients causing the cancer patient to waste away quickly. The major causes of cancer are stress, environmental factors, and diet. Research indicates that pancreatic and other enzymes are a vital part of a cancer program. It has also been noted that potassium is vital. Along with all the supplements, coffee enemas are important to cleanse the system and stimulate liver function.

(Beneficial Remedies, Treatments, and Nutrients)

HERBAL COMBINATION: (Red Clover Combination).

PHYSIOLOGIC ACTION: This herbal combination contains herbs that are very similar to the Hoxey formula used to treat cancer. It is unique in that it cleanses and feeds the body.

Note: Canaid herbal drink could be one of the cancer fighting breakthroughs that the world has so desperately been seeking. It's formula is similar, in nature and properties, to the famous Essiac treatment that has supposedly cured thousands of terminal cancer patients.

The herb Pau d' Arco possesses antibiotic, tumor inhibiting, virus killing, anti-fungal, and anti-malarial properties.

Red clover, burdock, and chaparral act as blood cleansers.

Single herbs: Bloodroot, Buckthorn Bark, Burdock, Chaparral, Cleavers, Garlic, Ginger, Ginseng, Golden Seal, Sheep Sorrel, Liquid Echinacea Extract, Pau d' Arco, Red Clover, Suma, Violet Leaves, and Yucca.

Also: There are various Chinese herbs which have been used successfully while treating cancer. Some of these herbs include: Reshi Mushroom, Astragalus, Ligustrum, Codonopsis, and Schizandra.

Vitamins: A, B3, B complex, C, E, Beta Carotene, Digestive Enzymes

Minerals: Germanium, Magnesium, Potassium, and Selenium.

Also: Almonds, Apricot Pits, Red Beet Juice, Liver Extract, Brewers Yeast, Raw Food, Low Animal Protein, Green Juices.

Helpful foods: Aloe Vera, apples, bananas, broccoli, bran, carrots, citrus fruits, green leafy vegetables, soybeans, sweet potatoes, turnip greens, vegetable oils, lean red meat, and fish liver oils.

CANDIDA ALBICANS (Candidiasis)

SPECIFICS: A yeast-like fungus that inhabits the genital tract, intestines, mouth, and throat. Candidiasis affects both men and women, when the fungus infects the vagina it results in vaginitis, when it infects the oral cavity, it is called thrush. Diabetics are at great risk of contracting the fungus, so if a person is diagnosed with yeast infection, he or she should be checked for diabetes.

(Beneficial Remedies, Treatments, and Nutrients)

HERBAL COMBINATION: (Cantrol).

PHYSIOLOGIC ACTION: An excellent well-balanced formula of herbs and supplements which balance the system while killing yeast. It includes caprylic acid and anti-oxidants for the control and eventual elimination of candida overgrowth.

Single herbs: Black Walnut, Caprinex, Garlicin, Pau d'Arco, and Yucca.

Vitamins: Biotin and B complex.

Also: Candida Cleanse, Yu-ccan, Caprylic Acid, Coenzyme Q10, L-Cysteine, Primadophilus, Primrose oil, and Salmon oil.

Helpful foods: Egg yolk, apricot, citrus fruits, beef kidney, beef liver, and vegetable and fish liver oils.

CANKER SORES

SPECIFICS: A canker sore is a contagious and painful mouth ulceration that can appear on the lips, gums, tongue, and on the inside cheeks. They are identified by a tingling sensation and a slight swelling of the mucous membrane. The sores have white centers and are surrounded by a red border. Canker sores may be caused from eating to many sweets, poor dental hygiene or stress.

(Beneficial Remedies, Treatments, and Nutrients)

Single herbs: Goldenseal, Pau d'Arco, and Burdock Root tea, or Red Raspberry tea is very helpful.

Vitamins: A, B5, B12, B complex, and large doses of C.

Minerals: Iron.

Also: Acidophilus and L-Lysine.

Note: Avoid chewing gum, sugar, processed or refined foods, and citrus fruits.

Helpful foods: Black molasses, carrots, lean red meat, fish, leafy green vegetables, turnips, potatoes, vegetable oils, and unpolished rice.

CARBUNCLES

SPECIFICS: A painful localized infection producing pus filled areas in the deeper layers of the skin tissues. Carbuncles are caused when bacteria enters lesions in the skin. They are deeper, slower healing and usually more painful than an ordinary boil.

(Beneficial Remedies, Treatments, and Nutrients)

HERBAL COMBINATION: (AKN).

PHYSIOLOGIC ACTION: AKN helps cleanse the bloodstream. Pimples, blackheads, and other superficial skin eruptions, and more serious conditions such as boils, carbuncles, dermatitis, eczema, and pleuritis will be eliminated when the blood has been cleansed.

Vitamins: A, B2, B3, B5, B6, C, F, P, Biotin, and Paba.

Minerals: Iron, Silicon, and Sulfur.

Also: Canaid herbal drink, Whey Powder, and Brewers Yeast.

Helpful foods: Almonds, apricots, avocados, beef, broccoli, black molasses, carrots, celery, flax seed, all fruits, safflower and linseed oil.

CARDIOVASCULAR DISEASE
(refer to Arteriosclerosis - page 14 and Circulation - page 43)

CARPAL TUNNEL SYNDROME

SPECIFICS: Carpal tunnel syndrome is a common nerve entrapment disorder caused by pressure on the median nerve at the point where it goes through the carpal tunnel of the wrist. This disorder is common in individuals who perform repetitive movements with their hands and wrist at work. It is characterized by pain, tingling, and burning sensations in the hand and fingers.

(Beneficial Remedies, Treatments, and Nutrients)

Single herbs: Ginger Root Caps.

Vitamins: B complex, plus B6, and C.

Minerals: Calcium and Magnesium.

Also: Bromelain.

Helpful foods: Kale, broccoli, green peppers, turnip greens, spinach, and pineapple.

CAR SICKNESS

SPECIFICS: Car sickness can indicate the presence of many diseases including inner ear infection, low blood sugar, food poisoning, and nutrient deficiency.

The most common cause is a deficiency of the vitamin "B6" and the mineral "magnesium". Ginkgo is excellent for chronic dizziness and light headedness.

(Beneficial Remedies, Treatments, and Nutrients)

HERBAL COMBINATION: (Motion Mate).

PHYSIOLOGIC ACTION: In a recent university study, ginger root caps proved more effective than either a drug or placebo at controlling motion induced nausea. Also queasy travelers have found taking B complex at night and just before the trip is most effective.

Single herbs: Ginger Root Caps and Ginkgo.

Vitamins: B complex, plus B6.

Minerals: Magnesium.

Helpful foods: Fruits, lean beef, nuts, unpolished rice, whole grains, and yellow corn.

CATARACTS

SPECIFICS: A cataract is a condition in which the lens of the eye becomes clouded or opaque, and unable to focus on close or far objects. Most cataracts are caused by free radical damage (exposure to low level radiation from x-rays and ultraviolet rays). Free radicals attack the structural enzymes, proteins, and cell membranes of the lens.

(Beneficial Remedies, Treatments, and Nutrients)

HERB COMPLEX: Cineraria Maritima, D3.

PHYSIOLOGIC ACTION: This product is a Homeopathic medicine and only available through your Homeopathic Doctor. Used regularly, this product will dissolve cataracts completely, after cataracts have disappeared use gencydo for minor inflammation.

HERBAL COMBINATION: (Herbal Eyebright Formula).

PHYSIOLOGIC ACTION: This herbal product contains valuable nutrients for the eyes. If taken regularly, in conjunction with a proper diet, cataracts are likely to dissolve.

Single herbs: Standardized Bilberry Extract.

Vitamins: A, B1, B2, B5, C, and E.

Minerals: Copper, Manganese, Selenium, and Zinc.

Also: L-Lysine neutralizes viruses, and is important in collagen formation, which is necessary for lens repair.

Helpful foods: Bran, beets, broccoli, carrots, green leafy vegetables, raisins, soybeans, sweet potatoes, vegetable oils, herring, and fish liver oils.

CELIAC DISEASE

SPECIFICS: Celiac disease is an intestinal disorder caused by the intolerance to a protein in wheat, barley, and rye called gluten. Treatment includes eating a well-balanced gluten-free diet, high in proteins, calories, and normal in fats. Exclude all cereal grains except corn and rice.

(Beneficial Remedies, Treatments, and Nutrients)

Vitamins: A, B6, B12, B complex, C, D, E, and K.

Minerals: Calcium, Iron, Magnesium, and Potassium.

Helpful foods: Apples, bananas, beets, black molasses, carrots, cheese, butter, goats milk, all fruit, kelp, and green leafy vegetables.

CERVICAL DYSPLASIA

SPECIFICS: A pre cancerous condition that occurs in the cervix of the female uterus. Cervical dysplasia is characterized by the presence of abnormal cells usually causing vaginal bleeding between menstrual periods and there may also be increased vaginal discharge. The (PAP) smear is most effective in diagnosing this condition.

(Beneficial Remedies, Treatments, and Nutrients)

Single herbs: Bloodroot and Calendula.

Vitamins: A, B complex, B6, B12, Folic acid, and C.

Minerals: Selenium and Zinc.

Also: Bitter orange oil, Bromelain, and Escarotic treatment.

Note: Avoid saturated fats from meat, white sugar, refined carbohydrates, and smoking.

Helpful foods: Greens, citrus fruits, strawberries, tomatoes, yellow fruits, and vegetables.

CHARLEY HORSE

SPECIFICS: A pulled or bruised muscle that results in soreness and stiffness caused by impaired blood circulation. It is usually caused by a forceful stretch of the leg during heavy exertion or athletic activity. Charley horse victims should have a protein rich diet to rebuild the damaged tissues.

(Beneficial Remedies, Treatments, and Nutrients)

HERBAL COMBINATION: (B F + C).

PHYSIOLOGIC ACTION: A special formula to aid in healing processes for torn cartilage's, sprained limbs, broken bones, multiple athletic injuries, and associated swelling and inflammation.

Single herbs: Comfrey Herb, Horsetail Grass, Oat Straw, Skullcap, and Yucca.

HOMEOPATHIC COMBINATION: Injury and Backache Formula.

Vitamins: B complex, B1, B2, B5, C, D, and E.

Minerals: Calcium, Magnesium, and Phosphorous.

Also: #12 tissue salts, Green-Lipid Mussel, Silica, Protein, and Unsaturated fatty acids.

Helpful foods: Red meat, butter, cheese, citrus fruits, soybeans, rice, sunflower seeds, nuts, whole grains, and sweet potatoes.

CHEMICAL ALLERGIES

SPECIFICS: The inappropriate response by the body's immune system to some foreign chemicals or environmental contaminants. The immune system wrongly identifies a toxic allergen causing the white blood cells to overreact creating more damage to the body than the allergen itself. Chemical allergies may cause asthma, diarrhea, dizziness, eczema, fever, hay fever, high blood pressure, hives, hypoglycemia, mental disorders, ringing in the ears, and stomach ulcers.

(Beneficial Remedies, Treatments, and Nutrients)

HERBAL COMBINATION: (HAS: Original and Fast Acting Formulas) (Allergy Care).

PHYSIOLOGIC ACTION: HAS is an excellent formula which contains herbs that help relieve symptoms of hay fever, sinus congestion, and respiratory allergies caused by chemicals. Helps drain nasal passages, relieve swollen membranes, eliminate mucus, and cleanse the body. The Fast Acting Formula adds Pseudoephedra, a natural plant extract from the Ephedra plant. This substance quickly opens nasal passages allowing free breathing. While HAS Fast Acting is not for prolonged use, HAS Original can be taken for as long as needed.

WARNING: Both formulas are not to be used during pregnancy, nor by small children.

Allergy Care: Maximum-strength natural allergy medicine that will not cause drowsiness. It contains 60mg of the active ingredient Pseudoephedrine Hcl.

Single herbs: Burdock Root, Cayenne, Chaparral, Elderberry, Eyebright, Lobelia, Golden Rod, Golden Seal, and Nettles

HOMEOPATHIC COMBINATION: Allergy Formula.

Vitamins: A, B complex plus extra B3, B6, C, and E.

Minerals: A multi-mineral complex plus Calcium, Magnesium, Manganese, and Potassium.

Also: Acidophilus, Bee Pollen, Coenzyme Q10, Germanium, L-Tyrosine, L-Cysteine, Digestive Enzymes, Pancreatic Enzymes, Propolis, Raw adrenal, and Raw thymus.

Helpful foods: Almonds, apples, beef, beets, broccoli, carrots, cheese, bananas, fruits, oat bran, safflower, and linseed oil.

CHICKEN POX

SPECIFICS: A highly contagious viral disease that first manifests as a fever and a mild headache. After twenty-four to thirty-six hours, the chief symptom is generalized skin eruptions. It is most important to keep infected children away from the elderly as the virus that causes chickenpox in children (Varicella Zoster) also causes shingles in adults.

(Beneficial Remedies, Treatments, and Nutrients)

HERBAL COMBINATION: (Fenu-Thyme) (ANT-PLG Syrup) (EchinaGuard).

PHYSIOLOGIC ACTION: Helps the body to resist infectious diseases and reduce fever. Acts as a support to the system during such illnesses as chicken pox, mumps, and measles.

Single herbs: Cayenne, Chickweed, Cleavers, Echinacea, Lobelia, and Red Clover.

Also: Canaid herbal drink strengthens the immune system. A bath can be made from bulk chickweed to alleviate itching. Chickweed ointment is also excellent for itching.

Vitamins: Complete multi-vitamin plus A, C, and E.

Minerals: Multi-mineral, plus Potassium, and Zinc.

Helpful foods: Bananas, citrus fruits, melon, herring, fish liver oils, carrots, broccoli, green leafy vegetables, sweet potatoes, and turnip greens.

CHOLESTASIS

SPECIFICS: Cholestasis is not in itself a disease, but a sign of a liver, kidney, or blood disorder, which causes a build-up of bilirubin in the blood. Bilirubin is the presence of pigments from worn out blood cells that are deposited in the tissues, which leads to a characteristic type of jaundice, causing the skin and whites of the eyes to become abnormally yellow.

(Beneficial Remedies, Treatments, and Nutrients)

HERBAL COMBINATION: (LG).

PHYSIOLOGIC ACTION: This herbal combination helps to correct malfunctioning of the liver and gall bladder. It is a liver detoxifier, and a bile stimulant.

Single herbs: Birch Leaves, Dandelion, Fennel, Horse Tail, Irish Moss, Parsley, and Rose Hips.

Vitamins: A, B6, C, D, and E.

Minerals: Calcium, Magnesium, and Phosphorus.

Also: Lecithin, Protein, and Unsaturated fatty acids.

Helpful foods: Apples, bananas, broccoli, carrots, cheese and other dairy products, tuna, fish liver oils, red meat, vegetable oils, and sprouted seeds.

Juices: Sauerkraut and tomato juice.

CHOLESTEROL LEVEL   (high)

SPECIFICS: Cholesterol is a fatty substance manufactured by the liver and found only in animal fat. It is essential in building sex hormones, cell membranes, and also aids in digestion. High cholesterol levels are the primary cause of heart disease and is implicated in clogging of the arteries, gall stones, high blood pressure, impotence, and mental impairment. High cholesterol can only be reduced by lowering ones consumption of low-density lipoproteins (LDLs - animal fats), eating a balanced diet, and exercise.

(Beneficial Remedies, Treatments, and Nutrients)

Single herbs: Cayenne, Garlic, Goldenseal, Hawthorn berries, Kelp, and Oat bran.

Vitamins: B complex, B3, B6, B9, B12, Choline, Inositol, C, and E.

Also: Coenzyme Q10, Guar Gum, Lecithin, and Lipotropic factors.

Helpful foods: Brewers yeast, broccoli, cabbage, spinach, fruit(citrus and other), fish liver oils, egg whites, vegetable oils, unpolished rice, and whole grains.

CHRONIC FATIGUE SYNDROME

SPECIFICS: Chronic fatigue syndrome is caused by the Epstein Barr virus (EBV). This virus is highly contagious and can be passed from one person to another by any close contact. The symptoms of chronic fatigue syndrome are anxiety, depression, extreme fatigue, irritability, headache, fever, swollen glands, sore throat, jaundice, and sleep disturbances.

(Beneficial Remedies, Treatments, and Nutrients)

Single herbs: Burdock root, Dandelion, Echinacea, Goldenseal, and Pau d'Arco.

Vitamins: Multi-vitamin complex plus A, B complex, B12, and E.

Minerals: Calcium, Magnesium, Potassium, Selenium, and Zinc.

Also: Acidophilus, Coenzyme Q10, Germanium, Protein, Proteolytic enzymes, and Raw thymus.

Helpful foods: Apples, aloe vera juice, bananas, citrus fruits, beef, bran, carrots, cheese, green leafy vegetables, herring, mushrooms, nuts, soybeans, and yams.

CHRONIC OBSTRUCTIVE LUNG DISEASE *(Refer to Emphysema - page 61)*

CIRCULATION

SPECIFICS: There are many disorders associated with circulatory problems. The most common disease for sluggish circulation is Raynaud's disease, characterized by constriction and spasm of the blood vessels in the limbs.

Poor circulation can also result from varicose veins, caused by the loss of elasticity in the walls of the veins. For information on high blood pressure refer to (arteriosclerosis) or (blood pressure high).

(Beneficial Remedies, Treatments, and Nutrients)

HERBAL COMBINATIONS: (H Formula) (Ginkgold).

PHYSIOLOGIC ACTION: Contains herbs which strengthen the heart and builds the vascular system. When taken with Cayenne, it improves circulation, giving a warming sensation to the entire body.

<u>Note:</u> Cayenne strengthens the pulse rate and circulation while Black Cohosh slows it down.

Single herbs: Cayenne, Black Cohosh, Bayberry, Butchers Broom, Ginkgo, and Yarrow.

Vitamins: A, B3, C, and E.

Minerals: Calcium, Magnesium, Potassium, and Selenium.

Also: Coenzyme Q10, Germanium, Lecithin, L-Carnitine, L-Cysteine, L-Methionine, and Multi-digestive enzymes.

Helpful foods: Alfalfa, beet, blackberry, grape, parsley, and pineapple juice.

CIRRHOSIS OF THE LIVER

SPECIFICS: A chronic degenerative, inflammatory, disease in which damage and hardening of the liver cells occur. Scarring of the liver cells renders the liver unable to function properly. The most common cause is excessive alcohol consumption. Other causes are malnutrition, chronic inflammation, and viral hepatitis. Damage from excessive drinking is irreversible, however further damage can be prevented by eating properly, abstaining from alcohol, and taking vitamin and mineral supplements.

(Beneficial Remedies, Treatments, and Nutrients)

Single herbs: Barberry, Burdock, Celandine, Dandelion, Echinacea, Fennel, Garlic, Goldenseal, Hops, Milk Thistle, Red Clover, and Suma.

Vitamins: A, B3, B9, B12, B complex, C, D, E, and K.

Minerals: Magnesium, and Zinc.

Also: Carbohydrates, Coenzyme Q10, L-Carnitine, L-Glutathionine, L-Methionine, and Protein.

Helpful foods: Apples, beef, butter, cheese, bran, broccoli, carrots, citrus fruits, green leafy vegetables, sardines, fish liver oils, and whole grains.

CLAP
(refer to Gonorrhea - page 76)

(refer to Gonorrhea - page 76)

COLD FEET

(Beneficial Remedies, Treatments, and Nutrients)

HERBAL COMBINATION: (Cayenne extract).

PHYSIOLOGIC ACTION: Improves pulse rate and circulation giving a warming sensation to the entire body.

Single herbs: Cayenne, Bayberry, and Kelp.

Vitamins: Vitamin E, and Niacin.

Minerals: A complete multi-mineral complex.

Helpful foods: Brewers yeast, kelp, soybeans, sunflower seeds, white meat of poultry, and vegetable oils.

COLDS AND COUGHS

SPECIFICS: A general inflammation of the mucous membranes of the respiratory passages caused by a virus. Symptoms include aches, pains, coughing, headache, fever, sneezing, congestion watery eyes, and difficult breathing.

(Beneficial Remedies, Treatments, and Nutrients)

HERBAL COMBINATIONS: (Fenu-Thyme) (Garlic Syrup) (Loquat Syrup) (Garlicin CF).

PHYSIOLOGIC ACTION: These herbal syrups and combinations work to soothe the throat and lungs and act as expectorants and demulcents to cut and expel mucus from the lungs. Garlicin CF is a unique formula combining the natural benefits of Garlic with other herbs such as Echinacea, Vitamin C, bioflavanoids, and Zinc.

Single herbs: Echinacea, Ginger, Pau d'Arco, and Yarrow.

HOMEOPATHIC COMBINATION: Dry Cough Formula.

Vitamins: Multi-vitamin complex plus C.

Minerals: Multi-mineral complex plus Zinc.

Also: Proteolytic enzymes, and Canaid herbal drink.

Helpful foods: Apples, citrus fruit, celery, herring, oysters, and turnip greens.

Juices: Apple, celery, and watercress.

COLDS AND FLU
(See Colds and Cough - page 45)

SPECIFICS: The flu is a highly contagious viral infection of the respiratory tract and is spread by coughing and sneezing. Symptoms include headache, fever, aching of limbs and back, and weakness.

(Beneficial Remedies, Treatments, and Nutrients)

HERBAL COMBINATIONS: (C+F) (Herbal Influence) (ANT-PLG Syrup).

PHYSIOLOGIC ACTION: Proven herbal formulas to help relieve symptoms of colds, flu, hoarseness, colic, cramps, sluggish circulation, beginning of fevers and germinal viral infections. Herbal Influence (formerly known as Herbal Composition) this formula was created by the early American herbalist, Samuel Thomson. It contains herbs which help with fever and nauseousness.

Single herbs: Cayenne, Red Clover, Raspberry Tea, Chaparral, Rose Hips, Garlic, Honey, and Golden Seal.

HOMEOPATHIC COMBINATION: Cold and Flu Formula.

Vitamins: A, B6, C, and P.

Minerals: Multi-mineral complex.

Also: Proteolytic enzymes and Canaid herbal drink.

Helpful foods: Apples, apricots, cherries, citrus fruits, lean beef, broccoli, carrots, green leafy vegetables, melon, nuts, sweet potatoes, turnip greens, and unpolished rice.

Juices: Apple, Carrot, Celery, Grapefruit, and Coconut juice.

COLD SORES *(Herpes Simplex Virus 1)*

SPECIFICS: Herpes simplex 1 results in cold sores and skin eruptions. They usually occur with a cold, fever, infection, or when the immune system is depressed. It can also cause inflammation of the eye. If the eye becomes infected see a doctor at once. By strengthening the immune system one can defend against or prevent herpes activation.

(Beneficial Remedies, Treatments, and Nutrients)

Single herbs: Echinacea, Goldenseal, Myrrh, and Red Clover.

Vitamins: B complex, C, and E.

Minerals: Zinc chelate.

Also: The amino acid L-Lysine has a direct effect on the virus.

Helpful foods: Herring, oysters, sardines, citrus fruits, red meats, and vegetable oils.

COLIC *(Infants)*

SPECIFICS: Colic most often occurs shortly after feeding. During an attack the baby suffers physical pain, gas, and cramps.

(Beneficial Remedies, Treatments, and Nutrients)

HERBAL COMBINATION: (Catnip and Fennel Extract).

PHYSIOLOGIC ACTION: This formula works on minor spasms, acid stomach and gas. It also soothes indigestion and nerves. Excellent for children.

Single herbs: Catnip, fennel, chamomile, peppermint or any combination in a tea. Make teas very mild. No sugar.

Note: Check your own diet if nursing baby.

HOMEOPATHIC COMBINATION: Colic Formula.

COLITIS

SPECIFICS: Mucous Colitis is often associated with, and made worse by psychological stress. Emotional upset should be avoided. Various herbs with multiple properties must be used to address the complexity of this situation.

Note: Avoid citrus juices. Bananas are very soothing and healing in ulcerative colitis. Primadophilus is effective in stabilizing flora in lower bowel.

(Beneficial Remedies, Treatments, and Nutrients)

Single herbs: Alfalfa, Bayberry, Chamomile, Caraway, Garlic, Reshi Mushroom, Plantain, Valerian, Wild Yam, and Yucca.

Vitamins: A, B6, Folic acid, Pantothenic acid, B complex, C, and E.

Minerals: Calcium, Iron, Magnesium, and Potassium.

Also: Multi-digestive and Proteolytic enzymes, Raw thymus glandular, and unsaturated fatty acids.

Helpful foods: Apples, bananas, lean beef, black molasses, tuna, fish liver oils, cheese, non citrus fruit, mushrooms, and sweet potatoes.

CONJUNCTIVITIS

SPECIFICS: An inflammation of the mucous membrane that lines the eyelids. The most common cause of conjunctivitis is a calcium deficiency, however a deficiency of vitamin A, B6, or riboflavin may cause conjunctivitis symptoms.

(Beneficial Remedies, Treatments, and Nutrients)

Vitamins: A, B2, B6, B complex, Niacin, C, and D.

Minerals: Calcium, Magnesium, and Phosphorus.

Helpful foods: Apricots, citrus fruits, cherries, beef, black molasses, broccoli, carrots, butter, cheese, shell fish, tuna, and whole wheat.

CONSTIPATION (Minor)

SPECIFICS: Constipation results when the waste material moves too slowly or there is decreased frequency of bowel movements. Constipation usually arises from insufficient amounts of fiber and fluids in the diet. Other causes include lack of exercise, nervousness, stress, infections, and poor diet.

(Beneficial Remedies, Treatments, and Nutrients)

HERBAL COMBINATION: (Multilax #1) or (Naturalax #1).

PHYSIOLOGIC ACTION: Helps relieve minor constipation.

WARNING: Do not use when abdominal pain nausea or vomiting are present. Frequent or prolonged use of preparation may result in dependence on laxatives.

Single herbs: Cascara Sagrada, Comfrey, Flaxseed, Goldenseal, Psyllium seed, Senna, and Yucca.

HOMEOPATHIC COMBINATION: Constipation and Hemorrhoids Formula.

Vitamins: A, B complex, C, D, and E.

Minerals: Calcium, Magnesium, Potassium, and Zinc.

Also: Yu-ccan herbal drink, Vita Cleansing Tea, Swiss Kriss, Metab Herb, Psyllium Husks, Flax meal, Super D Tea. Drink lots of pure water to flush system.

Helpful foods: Bananas, prunes, citrus fruits, all dairy products except cheese, carrots, turnips, green vegetables, soybeans, vegetable oils, and kelp.

Juices: Celery, Grapefruit, and Spinach juice.

CONSTIPATION (Chronic)

SPECIFICS: Chronic constipation is generally due to weakness of the muscles of the abdomen and the pelvic floor, which prevents adequate pressure when attempting to move the bowels. This condition is most prevalent in the elderly and persons with immobility problems.

(Beneficial Remedies, Treatments, and Nutrients)

HERBAL COMBINATIONS: (Multilax #2) or (Naturalax #2) (Laxacil) (Multilax 3) (Naturalax 3) (Aloelax Formula).

PHYSIOLOGIC ACTION: There are two forms of laxatives, stimulant and bulk forming. Stimulant laxatives encourage peristalsis of the bowel. This motion empties the intestinal tract of waste. Bulk forming laxatives absorb water and toxic wastes from the intestinal walls. The natural expansion triggers peristalsis, and pushes old fecal matter through the bowel. Both forms of laxatives have benefits.

WARNING: Most laxatives should not be taken during pregnancy. Psyllium husks, however, are safe.

Single herbs: Aloe Vera, Cascara Sagrada, Comfrey, Flaxseed, Goldenseal, Pepsin, Psyllium, Senna, and Yucca.

Vitamins: A, B1, B6, Choline, Inositol, Niacin, Pantothenic acid, B complex, C, D, and E.

Minerals: Calcium, Magnesium, Potassium, and Zinc.

BABIES: Licorice tea (made weakly). Nursing mothers can pass this one to the infant.

Also: Fats, Fiber, and Primadophilus.

Helpful foods: Same as minor constipation.

CONTACT DERMATITIS

SPECIFICS: Contact dermatitis is an allergy to something that touches the skin, that produces flaking, scaling, itching, and eventual thickening and color changes of the skin. The best way to cure this ailment is to remove the source of the allergen and cleanse the blood.

(Beneficial Remedies, Treatments, and Nutrients)

HERBAL COMBINATION: (AKN).

PHYSIOLOGIC ACTION: Many skin problems are related to liver dysfunction. This formula gives support to the liver, helps to cleanse the blood, and supplies nutrients for the skin.

Single herbs: Aloe Vera (on skin), Burdock, Cleavers, Dandelion, Evening Primrose, Garlic, Golden Seal, Pau d'Arco, Yellowdock, and Yucca.

Vitamins: A, B complex, B2, B3, B6, D, E, and Biotin B complex.

Minerals: Sulfur ointment, Potassium, and Zinc.

Also: Yu-ccan herbal drink, and Protein.

Helpful foods: Raw carrots, fish liver oils, green leafy vegetables, and vegetable oils.

CONVULSION
(Refer to Epilepsy - page 63)

COPPER TOXICITY

SPECIFICS: Copper is required by the body in minute amounts. This metallic element forms the essential part of several enzymes. Poisoning is usually due to people drinking home made alcohol distilled using copper tubing, using copper cookware, copper plumbing, and insecticides. Copper toxicity can lead to depression, nephritis, eczema, damage to the central nervous system, and sickle cell anemia.

(Beneficial Remedies, Treatments, and Nutrients)

Single herbs: Alfalfa and Garlic.

Vitamins: C.

Minerals: Calcium, Iron, Magnesium, Sulfur, and Zinc.

Also: L-Cysteiene, L-Lysine, and L-Methionine.

Helpful foods: Eggs, onions, pumpkin seeds, and other foods that have a high zinc content.

COUGHS

SPECIFICS: Refex action to try to clear the air-ways of mucus (phelegm) or other irritants or blockages. Most coughs are due to irritation of the airways by dust, gases, or smoke, or by mucus dripping from the back of the nose. An unproductive or dry cough does not bring up mucus or dry sputum.

(Beneficial Remedies, Treatments, and Nutrients)

HERBAL COMBINATIONS: (Fenu-Thyme) (Garlic Syrup) (Loquat Syrup) (Garlicin CF)

PHYSIOLOGIC ACTION: These herbal syrups and combinations work to soothe the throat and lungs and act as expectorants and demulcents to cut and expel mucus from the lungs. Garlicin CF is a unique formula combining the natural benefits of Garlic with other herbs such as Echinacea, Vitamin C, bioflavanoids and Zinc.

HERBAL TONICS: Pie Pa Koa, Salus, Olbas, Swiss herbal candy

HOMEOPATHIC COMBINATION: Dry Cough Formula.

Single herbs: Fenugreek Seed, Comfrey Leaves, Garlic, Rose Hips,

Vitamins: A, B6, C, and P.

Also: Honey, short fasts, and Zinc Lozenges.

Helpful foods: Apricot, apple, cherry, grape, and all citrus juices.

CRADLE CAP

SPECIFICS: A form of Siborrheic Dermatitis. A recurring condition, most prevalent in babies between the ages of three to nine months. Thick yellow scales occur in patches over the scalp and can also occur on the face, neck, and behind the ears. Cradle cap is harmless if the scalp does not become infected.

(Beneficial Remedies, Treatments, and Nutrients)

TREATMENT: Apply olive oil or vitamin E on the head and brush gently.

Also: A mild dandruff shampoo can be used.

CRAMPS

(Refer to "Leg Cramps" or "Menstrual Cramps")

CROHN'S DISEASE

SPECIFICS: A chronic and long-lasting inflammation of a section of the digestive tract. Inflammation works through all layers of the intestinal wall and involves the adjacent lymph nodes. If left untreated, it can increase the risk of cancer. The following nutrients are beneficial to the prevention and cure of this disease.

(Beneficial Remedies, Treatments, and Nutrients)

Single herbs: Echinacea, Garlic, Goldenseal, Pau d'Arco, Rose Hips, and Yerba Mate.

Vitamins: A strong multi-vitamin plus A, B12, B complex, and E.

Minerals: A complete mineral complex.

Also: Acidophlus, Aloe Vera, Essential fatty acids, and Protein.

CROUP

SPECIFICS: A respiratory infection that causes the larynx to swell, narrowing the air passage so the victim experiences difficulty breathing, tightness in the lungs, hoarseness, and a harsh high pitched cough.

Treatment involves a well-balanced diet and the following supplements to promote the growth and repair of tissues.

(Beneficial Remedies, Treatments, and Nutrients)

HERBAL COMBINATION: (Breath aid)(BRE).

PHYSIOLOGIC ACTION: This formula helps to restore free breathing by opening up the bronchial passages. It is especially effective for the shortness of breath, tightness of chest, and wheezing associated with croup.

Single herbs: Comfrey, Echinacea tincture, Fenugreek, and Goldenseal.

HOMEOPATHIC COMBINATION: Dry Cough Formula.

Vitamins: A, C, and E.

Minerals: Zinc.

Also: Cod liver oil, and Protein.

Juices: Apple, celery, grapefruit, and watercress.

CYSTIC FIBROSIS

SPECIFICS: A hereditary disease that begins during infancy, though symptoms may manifest themselves later in life.
This disease affects the endocrine, and exocrine glands. The victim experiences impaired gastrointestinal absorption, and recurrent lung infections. The greatest danger is malnutrition due to underproduction of digestive juices. The following nutrients are beneficial in the treatment of this disease.

(Beneficial Remedies, Treatments, and Nutrients)

Single herbs: Echinacea, Ginger, Goldenseal, and Yarrow.

Vitamins: A, B2, B6, Pantothenic acid, C, D, E, and K.

Minerals: Copper, Selenium, Sodium, and Zinc.

Also: Acidophlus, Coenzyme Q10, Germanium, Lecithin, Protein, Proteolytic enzymes, and Raw thymus.

Helpful foods: Aloe Vera, beef, bacon, bean, butter, broccoli, carrots, herring, oysters, fish liver oils, vegetable oils, and green leafy vegetables.

CYSTITIS
(refer to Kidney and Bladder - page 96)

DANDRUFF

SPECIFICS: A condition caused by dysfunctional sebaceous glands in the scalp. It can substantially be controlled by the use of B vitamin supplements and a diet of unrefined carbohydrates. A shampoo designed to control dandruff is also recommended.

(Beneficial Remedies, Treatments, and Nutrients)

Single herbs: Burdock, Chaparral, Red Clover, and Yarrow. May be used as teas or rubbed on the head.

Vitamins: A, B complex, B6, C, and E.

Minerals: Selenium, and Zinc.

Also: Unsaturated fatty acids.

Helpful foods: Bran, carrots, all fruits, lean beef, herring, oysters, nuts, and whole grains.

DEAFNESS
(refer to Ear Infections - page 59)

DECUBITUS ULCERS
(refer to Bed Sores - page 20)

DEPRESSION

SPECIFICS: The body can handle minor anxiety, but long term chronic depression and fatigue causes the body to break down. Long term depression occurs when the situation that causes anxiety is not relieved. Find the cause and handle it constructively. People experiencing depression should maintain a well-balanced diet and replace the nutrients depleted during anxiety or stress.

(Beneficial Remedies, Treatments, and Nutrients)

HERBAL COMBINATIONS: (Ginseng, Gotu Kola Plus) (Adren-Aid).

PHYSIOLOGIC ACTION: These excellent formulas build zest, energy, stamina, mental alertness, and reflex action. The herbs also help provide adrenal support which affect depression.

Single herbs: Bee Pollen, Cayenne, Damiana, Gotu Kola, St. John's Wort, Scullcap, Shitaki Mushroom, and Siberian Ginseng, and Yucca.

HOMEOPATHIC COMBINATION: Fatigue Formula.

Vitamins: B3, B6, B12, B complex(stress vitamin), lots of Vit C, plus a strong multi-vitamin.

Minerals: Mineral complex, plus Calcium, Chromium, Magnesium, and Zinc chelate.

Also: Bee pollen, Lithium, Primrose oil, Spirulina, L-Tryptophan and L-Tyrosine.

Helpful foods: Apples, broccoli, butter, cheese, citrus fruits, chicken, green leafy vegetables, sardines, shell fish, and whole grains.

DERMATITIS

SPECIFICS: An inflammatory, usually recurring skin reaction, that produces flaking, scaling, itching, and eventual thickening and color changes of the skin.

(Beneficial Remedies, Treatments, and Nutrients)

HERBAL COMBINATION: (AKN).

PHYSIOLOGIC ACTION: Many skin problems are related to liver dysfunction. This formula gives support to the liver, helps to cleanse the blood, and supplies nutrients for the skin.

Single herbs: Aloe Vera (on skin), Burdock, Cleavers, Dandelion, Evening Primrose, Garlic, Golden Seal, Pau d'Arco, Yellowdock, and Yucca.

Vitamins: A, B complex, B2, B3, B6, D, E, and Biotin B complex.

Minerals: Sulfur ointment, Potassium, and Zinc.

Also: Yu-ccan herbal drink, and Protein.

Helpful foods: Raw carrots, fish liver oils, green leafy vegetables, and vegetable oils.

DIABETES

SPECIFICS: Diabetes is the result of insufficient production of insulin by the pancreas. Insulin is a hormone that is essential for the conversion of glucose into energy. The resulting symptoms range in severity from mental confusion to coma. Generally a well-balanced diet, rich in vitamins and minerals, is one of the most important factors in the control of diabetes.

(Beneficial Remedies, Treatments, and Nutrients)

HERBAL COMBINATION: (PC).

PHYSIOLOGIC ACTION: An excellent formula to stimulate and restore natural functions of the pancreas and spleen. Contains a natural form of insulin thus relieving most symptoms associated with diabetes.

Single herbs: Buchu, Dandelion, Cayenne, Cedar Berries, Goldenseal, Licorice Root, Mullein, Suma, Juniper and Uva Ursi.

Vitamins: A, B complex, B1, B2, B6, B12, Choline, Inositol 89 E, and P.

Minerals: Calcium, Chromium, Iron, Potassium, Magnesium, and Zinc.

Also: Lecithin, Protein, and Proteolytic enzymes.

Helpful foods: Apricots, bananas, beef, chicken, blackstrap molasses, butter, cheese, herring, oysters, carrots, turnip greens, and soybeans.

DIAPER RASH

SPECIFICS: Quite similar to a heat rash. Caused by infrequent changing of diapers or undergarments. Massage the affected area daily is very helpful. Frequent sponge baths with warm water and a mild herbal soap or a soap containing vitamin E are recommended.

(Beneficial Remedies, Treatments, and Nutrients)

HERBAL OINTMENTS: (X-Itch ointment) (Derm-Aid Ointment).

Single herbs: Mullein Leaf and Slippery Elm (used internally in juice or apply as paste).

Vitamins: Mom can take Vitamins A, B, and C.

Also: Vitamin E, Powdered Golden Seal, or Comfrey added to baby powder.

DIARRHEA

SPECIFICS: A condition causing frequent elimination of loose watery stools. Because of the rapid expulsion of food through the lower digestive tract, the victim does not properly absorb nutrients and can therefore develop nutrient deficiencies. Treatment for diarrhea includes a diet rich in protein, vitamins, and minerals.

(Beneficial Remedies, Treatments, and Nutrients)

HERBAL COMBINATION: (Diarid).

PHYSIOLOGICAL ACTION: This is a maximum-strength formula that relieves diarrhea and the pain and cramping that accompany it. The active ingredient is called Activated Attapulgite, a special kaolin substance with water absorbing abilities.

Single herbs: Blackberry Root, Red Raspberry, Slippery Elm, and Yucca.

HOMEOPATHIC COMBINATION: Indigestion & Gas Formula.

Vitamins: A, B complex, B1, B2, B3, B6, C, Folic acid, and Choline.

Minerals: Calcium, Chlorine, Iron, Magnesium, Potassium, and Sodium.

Also: Nutmeg and Cloves for cramps, Acidophilus, Activated Charcoal, and Digestive enzymes.

BABIES and CHILDREN: Slippery Elm enema, Red Raspberry tea, fresh apple juice, banana, brown rice water, or carob.

Juices: Carrot and Blackberry juice.

DIGESTIVE DISORDERS *(Dyspepsia)*

SPECIFICS: Dyspepsia is a disorder in the stomach or small or large intestine usually caused by the fermentation of food in the colon, producing carbon dioxide and hydrogen. Symptoms include abdominal pain, belching, gas, heartburn, nausea, bloating, and vomiting.

(Beneficial Remedies, Treatments, and Nutrients)

HERBAL COMBINATIONS: (Multilax #2) or (Naturalax #2).

PHYSIOLOGIC ACTION: Helps intestinal gas, indigestion, heartburn, and stomach ache. Warm Peppermint tea, Cayenne, Papaya, or Aloe Vera can be taken with meals.

Single herbs: Aloe Vera, Chamomile, Cayenne, Comfrey leaves, Fennel, Ginger, Golden Seal, Licorice, Marshmallow Root, Papaya, and Yucca.

HOMEOPATHIC COMBINATION: Indigestion & Gas Formula.

Vitamins: A, B3, B complex, and Biotin.

Minerals: Copper, Dolomite, Iodine, Phosphorus, Potassium, and Zinc.

Also: Digestive Enzymes, Garlic, Bee Pollen, Calmus Root tea, Lactic Acid foods, Swedish Bitters, Primadophilus, and Yu-ccan.

Helpful foods: Avocados, bananas, red meat, bacon, chicken, cheese, oat bran, and whole grains.

DIVERTICULITIS

SPECIFICS: Diverticulitis is when the colon's mucous membranes become inflamed, resulting in the formation of small sacs (diverticula), that may be found along the small or large intestine. In very severe cases the disease can result in perforation of the colon, causing severe bleeding.

(Beneficial Remedies, Treatments, and Nutrients)

HERBAL COMBINATION: (Naturalax or Multilax #2).

PHYSIOLOGIC ACTION: The most effective prevention for diverticulitis is to avoid constipation. The above combination both tones and naturally accelerates internal cleansing of the body through the bowels. This combination acts as a tonic to the entire digestive system, it strengthens the tissue of the intestinal tract, resulting in a healthier muscular reaction.

WARNING: Do not take during pregnancy!

Single herbs: Alfalfa, Cayenne, Chamomile, Garlic, Papaya, Psyllium, Red Clover, and Yarrow.

Vitamins: A, B complex, C, E, and K.

Minerals: Multi-mineral

Also: Fiber (Oat bran, Glucomannan), Multi-digestive and Proteolytic enzymes, and Acidophlus.

Helpful foods: Broccoli, carrots, celery, corn, fish liver oils, all sea foods, citrus fruits, pineapples, and nuts.

Juices: Celery and spinach juice

DROPSY

SPECIFICS: Dropsy is caused by fluid accumulation in the body. The retention of fluids appears as swelling and is often seen in the hands and feet, but may be located in any area of the body. Fluid retention is often caused by allergies.

(Beneficial Remedies, Treatments, and Nutrients)

HERBAL COMBINATION: (KB).

PHYSIOLOGIC ACTION: KB acts as a mild diuretic to rid the body of excessive water. Disorders that cause edema are sodium retention, congestive heart failure, weak kidneys, varicose veins, and protein and thiamine deficiencies.

Single herbs: Alfalfa, Buchu, Dandelion tea, Juniper, lobelia, Parsley, Pau d'Arco tea, Safflower, Uva Ursi, and Yarrow.

Vitamins: B1, B6, B complex, C, D, and E.

Minerals: Calcium, Copper, and Potassium.

Also: L-Taurine, #9 and #11 tissue salts, Silicon, low Sodium, and Protein.

Helpful foods: All sea foods, red meats, chicken, cheese, fruits(citrus and other), soybeans, spinach, sprouted seeds, and whole grains.

DRUG DEPENDENCY

SPECIFICS: A chronic physiological or psychological condition marked by a dependence on drugs. Deficiencies of many nutrients occur when taking drugs. Some effects of drugs are a depressed immune system, damage to the central nervous system, brain, duodenum, pancreas, liver, and a loss of inhibition.

Note: Tobacco, alcohol, caffeine and other drug "cravings" are brought about by a physiological body dependence on the poison which develops during prolonged use. The addicts blood poison level must remain at a certain level at all times. As the poison level drops, there is a "desire" to take in more of the drug, to bring the level back again.

(Beneficial Remedies, Treatments, and Nutrients)

HERBAL COMBINATIONS: (AdrenAid) (Red Clover Comb).

PHYSIOLOGIC ACTION: These herbal formulas provide support to the body while cleansing toxins. Red Clover Combination will minimize withdrawal symptoms such as headache, insomnia, sensitivity to light, irrational thinking, disorientation, and should be used with all detoxification programs.

Single herbs: Pau d'Arco, Chamomile tea, Licorice Root, and Lobelia.

Vitamins: B complex, and C.

Minerals: Calcium, and Potassium.

Also: Tyrosine, Vitamins B, C, and E, alleviates depression, fatigue, and irritability when dependent on cocaine, hashish, and marijuana.

Refer to: "Note in SMOKING" in this manual.

Helpful foods: All fruits, red meats, chicken, honey, seafood's, nuts, raw vegetables, and vegetable oils.

DYSMENORRHEA

SPECIFICS: Dysmenorrhea is associated with the hormonal changes in teenage girls and young women. Symptoms consist of pain, bloated abdomen, cramps, and discomfort during or just before a menstrual period. The best prevention for Dysmenorrhea is a nutrient rich diet, supplemented with vitamins and minerals, plus a good exercise program.

(Beneficial Remedies, Treatments, and Nutrients)

HERBAL COMBINATIONS: (FC) or (FEM-MEND).

PHYSIOLOGIC ACTION: Helps regulate the menstrual cycle, relieve cramps, bloating, and strengthens and regulates the kidneys, bladder and uterus areas. Beneficial for all female and uterine complaints.

WARNING: Do not use this combination while taking estrogen or oral contraceptives!

Single herbs: Dong Quai, Kelp, Red Raspberry, and Uva Ursi.

Vitamins: B complex, B5, B6, B12, C, E, and K.

Minerals: Calcium, Chlorine, Chromium, Iodine, Iron, Magnesium, and Manganese.

Also: Inositol, L-Lysine, L-Tyrosine, Methionine, Spirulina, and Primrose oil.

Helpful foods: All vegetables and vegetable oils, fish and fish liver oils, cheese, butter, apples, bananas, citrus fruits, and mushrooms.

DYSPEPSIA
(refer to Digestive Disorders - page 56)

EAR INFECTIONS

SPECIFICS: The most common type of ear infection is outer ear infection(otitis externa). Symptoms of the infection are fever, severe pain, and discharge from the ear. Middle ear infections(otitis media) are common in children and are usually caused by the spread of bacteria from the nose and throat. Symptoms include pressure in the ear and earache. Infection in the inner ear is usually caused by the spread of bacteria from a middle ear infection. Symptoms include fever, loss of hearing, dizziness, and vomiting.

(Beneficial Remedies, Treatments, and Nutrients)

HERBAL COMBINATIONS: (ImmunAid) (B&B Extract) (EchinaGuard).

PHYSIOLOGIC ACTION: ImmunAid boosts immunity, thereby helping with ear infections. EchinaGuard is a liquid and Echinacea extract is excellent for small children with ear infections. B&B Extract can be placed in the ear or taken internally. It is also used to aid poor equilibrium, and nervous conditions.

Single herbs: Blue Cohosh, Echinacea, Garlic Oil, Garlic, Mullein Oil, Mullein, Skullcap, Sheep Sorrel, and St. Johns Wort.

HOMEOPATHIC COMBINATION: Earache Formula.

Vitamins: A, B complex, and C.

Minerals: Calcium and Zinc.

Also: Canaid herbal drink, Propolis, Protein, and Primadophilus. When combating ear infections, it is imperative to exclude allergen foods from the diet. This is particularly true of all dairy products.

Helpful foods: Lean red meat, carrots, green vegetables, citrus fruits, fish liver oils, herring, oysters, sardines, nuts, sprouted seeds, and sunflower seeds.

ECZEMA

SPECIFICS: A type of skin eruption characterized by tiny blisters that weep and crust. Chronic forms produce flaking, scaling, itching, and eventual thickening and color changes of the skin.

(Beneficial Remedies, Treatments, and Nutrients)

HERBAL COMBINATION: (AKN).

PHYSIOLOGIC ACTION: When toxins are not properly eliminated from the body, they may surface through the skin creating eczema. This formula has been created to support liver and gall bladder function, to ensure toxins are filtered from the blood.

Single herbs: Aloe Vera, Chickweed, Evening Primrose Oil, Pau d'Arco, Red Clover, Thisilyn (Milk Thistle), and Yellow Dock.

Vitamins: A, B complex, C, D, Paba, Biotin, Choline, and Inositol.

Minerals: Magnesium, Sulfur Ointment, and Zinc ointment.

Helpful foods: Apples, apricots, cherries, citrus fruits, all sea foods, lean red meat, chicken, broccoli, carrots, celery, vegetable oils, and grain sprouts.

Juices: Carrot, Celery, and Lemon juice.

Note: This condition is aggravated by food allergens such as dairy and wheat. These foods should be avoided. Powders and pastes should not be applied during acute or weeping stages. After acute stage passes, ointments and salves may be applied. Herbal ointments which contain Chickweed and Calendula are particularly helpful.

EDEMA

SPECIFICS: Edema is a fluid accumulation in the body. The retention of fluids appears as swelling and is often seen in the hands and feet, but may be located in any area of the body. Fluid retention is often caused by allergies.

(Beneficial Remedies, Treatments, and Nutrients)

HERBAL COMBINATION: (KB).

PHYSIOLOGIC ACTION: KB acts as a mild diuretic to rid the body of excessive water. Disorders that cause edema are sodium retention, congestive heart failure, weak kidneys, varicose veins, and protein and thiamine deficiencies.

Single herbs: Alfalfa, Buchu, Dandelion tea, Juniper, lobelia, Parsley, Pau d'Arco tea, Safflower, Uva Ursi, and Yarrow.

Vitamins: B1, B6, B complex, C, D, and E.

Minerals: Calcium, Copper, and Potassium.

Also: L-Taurine, #9 and #11 tissue salts, Silicon, low Sodium, and Protein.

Helpful foods: Fruit(citrus and other), beef, butter, cheese, egg whites, seafood, fish liver oils, broccoli, spinach, flax seed, and sunflower seeds.

EMPHYSEMA

SPECIFICS: Emphysema is caused by loss of elasticity and dilation of the lung tissue, resulting in abnormal swelling and destruction of the tiny air sacs of the lungs. Factors that contribute to the onset of emphysema are asthma, bronchitis, cigarette smoking, and exposure to air pollution.

(Beneficial Remedies, Treatments, and Nutrients)

HERBAL COMBINATIONS: (Breath-Aid) (BronCare) (Garlicin CF).

PHYSIOLOGICAL ACTION: These natural formulas help to restore free breathing by dilating bronchial passages. They also offer nutritional support to the lungs.

Single herbs: Anise Seed Oil, Comfrey, Elecampane, Fenugreek, Garlic, Lobelia, Mullein, and Swedish Bitters.

Vitamins: A, B complex, C, D, E, and Folic Acid.

Also: L-Cysteine, L-Methionine, Protein supplement, Multienzymes and Proteolytic enzymes.

Helpful foods: All dairy products, beef, chicken, black molasses, citrus fruits, carrots, green leafy vegetables, turnip tops, soybeans, and whole rye.

ENDOMETRIOSIS

SPECIFICS: Endometriosis is the condition of having uterine tissue in abnormal locations. The location of this uterine tissue is around the ovaries, fallopian tubes, rectum and peritoneum. Symptoms are pain in the lower back, abdomen, uterus and other pelvic organs, painful menstruation, and the passage of large clots and shreds of tissue during menses. High fat diets and genetics have been associated with the development of endometriosis.

(Beneficial Remedies, Treatments, and Nutrients)

Single herbs: Black Cohosh, Blue Cohosh, Chaste Tree, Dong Quai, Peony Root, Red Raspberry.

Vitamins: A, Beta-carotene, B complex, B6, C, and E.

Minerals: Calcium and Magnesium.

Also: Omega-3 and Omega-6 oils.

Helpful foods: All fresh water fish and vegetable oils.

ENTERITIS

SPECIFICS: A chronic and long-lasting inflammation of a section of the digestive tract. Inflammation works through all layers of the intestinal wall and involves the adjacent lymph nodes. If left untreated, it can increase the risk of cancer. The following nutrients are beneficial to the prevention and cure of this disease.

(Beneficial Remedies, Treatments, and Nutrients)

Single herbs: Echinacea, Garlic, Goldenseal, Pau d'Arco, Rose Hips, and Yerba Mate.

Vitamins: A strong multi-vitamin plus A, B12, B complex, and E.

Minerals: A complete mineral complex.

Also: Acidophlus, Aloe Vera, Essential fatty acids, and Protein.

ENTEROBIASIS
(refer to Parasites - page 126)

EPILEPSY

SPECIFICS: A disease characterized by seizures, caused by electrical disturbances in the nerve cells in one section of the brain. The epileptic should maintain a well-balanced diet and avoid all refined sugars, completely eliminate all animal proteins, except milk, as they rob body of magnesium and Vitamin B6 reserves. Eat lots of raw vegetables and fruit. Epileptics require plenty of fresh air, exercise and sound sleep.

(Beneficial Remedies, Treatments, and Nutrients)

HERBAL COMBINATION: (B&B Tincture).

PHYSIOLOGICAL ACTION: The herbs in this formula have a beneficial effect on the autonomic nervous system. It helps to calm the nerves and relax the muscles.

Single herbs: Black-Cohosh, Horse Nettle, Hyssop, Irish Moss, Mistletoe, and Skullcap.

Vitamins: A, B complex, Niacin, B6, B15, C, D, and E.

Minerals: Calcium, Chromium, Iron, and Magnesium.

Also: Germanium, L-Taurine, L-Tyrosine, Proteolytic enzymes, and Digestive enzymes.

Helpful foods: Apples, apricots, bananas, cherries, grapes, melon, citrus fruits, broccoli, carrots, celery, cauliflower, green peppers, and spinach.

EPSTEIN BARR VIRUS
(refer to Fatigue, Stress "Chronic" - page 64)

EXFOLIATION

SPECIFICS: An inflammatory, usually recurring skin reaction, that produces flaking, scaling, itching, and eventual thickening and color changes of the skin.

(Beneficial Remedies, Treatments, and Nutrients)

HERBAL COMBINATION: (AKN).

PHYSIOLOGIC ACTION: Many skin problems are related to liver dysfunction. This formula gives support to the liver, helps to cleanse the blood, and supplies nutrients for the skin.

Single herbs: Aloe Vera (on skin), Burdock, Cleavers, Dandelion, Evening Primrose, Garlic, Golden Seal, Pau d'Arco, Yellowdock, and Yucca.

Vitamins: A, B complex, B2, B3, B6, D, E, and Biotin B complex.

Minerals: Sulfur ointment, Potassium, and Zinc.

Also: Yu-ccan herbal drink, and Protein.

Helpful foods: Raw carrots, fish liver oils, green leafy vegetables, and vegetable oils.

EYE DISORDERS

SPECIFICS: A deficiency of any one of the vitamins can lead to eye problems. Most eye problems can be prevented by supplementing the diet with vitamins and the nutrients listed.

(Beneficial Remedies, Treatments, and Nutrients)

HERBAL COMBINATION: (Herbal Eye bright Formula).

PHYSIOLOGIC ACTION: Extremely valuable in strengthening and healing the eyes. Aids the body in healing lesions and eye injuries.

WARNING: If symptoms persist, discontinue use.

Note: The herb eye bright may be used as a wash for superficial inflammations of the eye.

Single herbs: Bilberry, and Eyebright.

Vitamins: A Multi-vitamin complex, plus A, B1, B2, B3, B5, B6, C D, and E.

Minerals: Calcium, Copper, Manganese, Magnesium, Potassium, Selenium, and Zinc.

Also: Gyncydo, and Protein.

Helpful foods: Apples, citrus fruits, beets, rice bran, carrots, green leafy vegetables, herring, oysters, red meat, chicken, nuts, and soybeans.

FARMERS LUNG
(refer to Allergies - page 9)

FATIGUE, STRESS (Chronic)

SPECIFICS: The body can handle minor stress but long term stress causes the body to break down. Fatigue occurs when the situation that causes stress is not relieved. Find the cause and handle it constructively. People experiencing depression should maintain a well-balanced diet and replace the nutrients depleted during anxiety or stress.

(Beneficial Remedies, Treatments, and Nutrients)

HERBAL COMBINATIONS: (AdrenAid) (Echinacea Astragalus and Reshi Combination) (ImmuneAid) (Healthy Greens).

PHYSIOLOGIC ACTION: The herbs in these combinations work to support the adrenal glands and act as a tonic boost to the immune system.

Single herbs: Astragalus, Cayenne, Echinacea, Ginkgo Bilobia, Siberian Ginseng, Ginseng, Gota Kola, Lobelia, Reshi Mushroom, Yucca, and all deep green herbs such as Barley Grass, Chlorella, Spirulina, and Garlic.

HOMEOPATHIC COMBINATION: Fatigue Formula.

Vitamins: A, Ester C with Bioflavonoids, B complex (high potency), E, D, and folic acid.

Minerals: Iron, Magnesium, Manganese, Potassium, Selenium, and Zinc.

Also: Canaid and Yu-ccan herbal drinks, Coenzyme Q 10, Fiber, and Raw Thymus.

Helpful foods: All fruits(citrus and other), black molasses, butter, cheese, beef, tuna, sardines, fish liver oils, beets, broccoli, carrots, vegetable oils, green leafy vegetables, soybeans, and sunflower seeds.

<u>FATIGUE</u> (Chronic)

SPECIFICS: Recent studies have shown that a combination of Evening Primrose Oil, and Fish Oil is very beneficial in combating chronic fatigue. The original study was called, "Efamol Marine." This product is not available in the United States nor Canada. It can be replicated by combining the individual Evening Primrose Oil capsules with Fish Oil, or Fish Liver Oil.

(Beneficial Remedies, Treatments, and Nutrients)

HERBAL COMBINATIONS: AdrenAid, Echinacea Astragalus and Reshi Combination, ImmuneAid, and Healthy Greens.

PHYSIOLOGICAL ACTION: The herbs in these combs. work to support the adrenal glands and acts as a tonic to the immune system

Single herbs: Astragalus, Echinacea, EchinaGuard Liquid Extract, Siberian Ginseng, Reshi Mushroom, Yucca, and all deep green herbs such as Barley Grass, Chlorella, Spirulina, & Garlic.

Vitamins: Ester C with Bioflavonoids, B Complex, E, & D.

Minerals: Calcium, Magnesium, Potassium, Selenium, & Zinc.

Also: CoQ 10, and Raw Thymus.

Helpful foods: Refer to Fatigue, Stress (chronic).

FATIGUE(General)

SPECIFICS: General fatigue is characterized by the feeling of mental and physical weariness usually caused by a nutrient deficiency or physical exertion.

(Beneficial Remedies, Treatments, and Nutrients)

HERBAL COMBINATION: (Herbal UP) (Energizer) (AdrenAid).

PHYSIOLOGIC ACTION: These herbal formulas combine herbs which support the adrenals, tonify the system, and offer stamina and endurance. Many of the herbs in these formulas are used by athletes to improve performance.

Single herbs: Siberian Ginseng, Gotu Kola, and Bee Pollen.

HOMEOPATHIC COMBINATION: Fatigue Formula.

Vitamins: Multi-vitamin and Mineral supplement, B Complex, B 12, and Vitamin C.

Minerals: GTF Chromium, Potassium, Selenium, and Zinc.

Helpful foods: Beef, chicken, herring, oysters, shellfish, all fruits, melon, raw vegetables, sweet potatoes, turnip greens, and unpolished rice.

FEVER BLISTERS
(Refer to Cold Sores - page 46)

FEVER and FLU COMPLAINTS

SPECIFICS: Fever is any temperature above that which is normal for the individuals body. The flu is a highly contagious viral infection of the respiratory tract and is spread by coughing and sneezing. Symptoms include headache, fever, aching of limbs and back, and weakness.

(Beneficial Remedies, Treatments, and Nutrients)

HERBAL COMBINATIONS: (Fenu-Thyme) (Herbal Influence) (Immune Aid).

PHYSIOLOGIC ACTION: These effective formulas help to cleanse toxins, combat infections and inflammations especially in the

lymphatic system. They give support to the immune system enabling the body to combat the illness.

HOMEOPATHIC COMBINATION: Cold and Flu Formula.

Vitamins: A, B complex, B1, B3, C, E, and P.

Minerals: Calcium, Phosphorus, Potassium, and Sodium.

Also: Canaid herbal drink, Cold Care, Propolis, Red Raspberry, Elder Flowers, Garlic, Rosehip, Golden Seal, Yarrow, Red Clover, #4 tissue salts.

Catnip and Peppermint together at onset of flu.

INFANTS and CHILDREN: Red Raspberry or Peppermint tea.

Helpful foods: Apricots, bananas, citrus fruits, broccoli, carrots, celery, corn, green leafy vegetables, bacon, beef, chicken, and fish liver oils.

Juices: Celery, grapefruit, lemon, and parsley juice.

FIBROCYSTIC DISEASE
OF THE BREAST

SPECIFICS: In fibrocystic disease, round cysts either firm or soft that move freely are produced. The cysts become filled with fluid, fibrous tissue encircles the cysts and thickens, forming a firm lump. The most common cause of this disease is iron deficiency. Other factors include hormone imbalance and abnormal breast milk production.

(Beneficial Remedies, Treatments, and Nutrients)

Single herbs: Echinacea, Goldenseal, Squaw vine, Mullein, Pau d'Arco, and Red Clover.

Vitamins: A, B1, B6, B complex, and C.

Minerals: A comprehensive multi-mineral formula.

Also: Coenzyme Q10, Germanium, and Proteolytic enzymes.

Helpful foods: Black molasses, fish liver oils, red meat, all fruits, nuts, and vegetables.

FLATULENCE

(refer to Digestive Disorders - page 56)

FLATWORM

SPECIFICS: Flatworms live in the gastrointestinal tract. Early signs include diarrhea, loss of appetite, and rectal itching. If not eliminated they will result in the loss of weight, colon disorders, and anemia. Causes include ingestion of eggs or larvae from partially cooked meat and improper disposal of human waste.

(Beneficial Remedies, Treatments, and Nutrients)

HERBAL COMBINATIONS: (Para-X) (Para-VF).

PHYSIOLOGIC ACTION: Useful in destroying and eliminating parasites, such as worms. Also helps relieve many kinds of skin problems. The Para-VF is a liquid and is useful for children and the elderly who cannot swallow capsules.

WARNING: Do not use during pregnancy!

Single herbs: Black Walnut, Garlic, Pumpkin Seeds, Sage, Swedish Bitters, and Wormwood.

Vitamins: Folic Acid.

Minerals: Iron and Zinc.

CHILDREN: Chamomile tea or raisins soaked in Senna tea for older children may be helpful.

Helpful foods: Asparagus, brewers yeast, broccoli, lettuce, lima beans, liver, mushrooms, nuts, and spinach.

FOOD ALLERGIES
(refer to Allergies - page 9)

FOOD POISONING

SPECIFICS: When a person consumes food containing harmful bacteria or viruses. Symptoms for common food poisoning include cramps, diarrhea, nausea, and vomiting.

(Beneficial Remedies, Treatments, and Nutrients)

Single herbs: Pau d'Arco.

Vitamins: C and E.

Minerals: Multi-mineral complex.

Also: Acidophlus, L-Cysteine, L-Methionine and Fiber.

Helpful foods: Bran, broccoli, soybeans, spinach, sweet potatoes, turnip greens, citrus fruits, vegetable oils, and whole wheat.

FRACTURE *(Broken Bone)*

SPECIFICS: A fracture is called "simple" when the skin remains intact and "open" when the broken bone protrudes through the skin.

(Beneficial Remedies, Treatments, and Nutrients)

HERBAL COMBINATION: (BF + C).

PHYSIOLOGIC ACTION: A special formula to aid the body's healing processes involved with broken bones, athletic injuries, sprained limbs, and related inflammation and swelling. A tonic used after acute and chronic diseases to help rebuild the body.

Single herbs: Comfrey Root, Black Walnut, Horsetail, Kelp, Lobelia, Skullcap, and White Oak Bark.

HOMEOPATHIC COMBINATION: Injury and Backache Formula.

Vitamins: A, Pantothenic acid, C, and D.

Minerals: Calcium, Magnesium, and Potassium.

Also: Silicon and Protein.

Helpful foods: Apples, bananas, citrus fruits, butter, cheese, and other dairy products, raw vegetables, vegetable oils, fish liver oils, flax seed, nuts, and sprouts.

<u>*Note:*</u> Avoid the consumption of red meat and products containing caffeine. Phosphorus can lead to bone loss, so preserved foods should be limited due to their high phosphorus content.

FRIGIDITY

SPECIFICS: The lack of desire for or inability to become aroused during sexual intercourse. Frigidity may be psychological or organic in nature. A balanced diet is important. Do not consume animal fats, fried foods, junk foods, or sugar!

(Beneficial Remedies, Treatments, and Nutrients)

HERBAL COMBINATION: (APH).

PHYSIOLOGIC ACTION: Stimulates male and female sexual impulses as well as strengthens and increases sexual power and helps fight fatigue.

Single herbs: Damiana, Ginkgo, Ginseng and Gotu Kola.

Vitamins: E, Paba, Folic acid, and Lecithin.

Minerals: Zinc, Iodine, and Calcium.

Also: L-Arginine, L-Tyrosine, Proteolytic enzymes, Melbrosia (for men), Tropical Impulse tea, Loving Mood, Bee pollen, Sesame seeds, and Ginseng.

Helpful foods: High quality vegetable oil, fertile eggs, raw milk.
Juices: Celery and parsley juice.

FUNGUS INFESTATIONS
(Athletes foot, ringworm, thrush)

SPECIFICS: Fungus infestations are highly contagious and live off dead skin cells. Victims of fungus infestations should eat a well-balanced diet, supplemented by megadoses of vitamins A, B, and C.

(Beneficial Remedies, Treatments, and Nutrients)

Single herbs: Black Walnut, Garlic, Caprinex, and Pau d'Arco.

Vitamins: A, B, C, and E.

Also: Primadophilus.

Helpful foods: Beef, chicken, tuna, carrots, black walnut, raw fruits, spinach, turnip greens, and sweet potatoes.

<u>Note:</u> Avoid dairy products and processed foods.

GALLBLADDER DISORDERS

SPECIFICS: The gallbladder is a small pear shaped organ located directly under the liver that contains bile. When this organ becomes inflamed, the person suffers severe pain in the right abdomen, accompanied by nausea and vomiting. Too much refined carbohydrate or too little protein in the diet prevents adequate bile production.

(Beneficial Remedies, Treatments, and Nutrients)

HERBAL COMBINATION: (KB).

PHYSIOLOGIC ACTION: Extremely valuable in healing and strengthening the kidneys, bladder and genito-urinary area. Useful to stop bed-wetting, but is a diuretic when congestion of the kidneys is indicated. Helps remove bladder, uterine and urethral toxins.

WARNING: Intended for occasional use only. May cause green-yellow discoloration of urine.

Single herbs: Alfalfa, Barberry root, Catnip, Dandelion, Fennel, Ginger root, Horsetail, and Wild Yam.

Vitamins: A, B complex, Choline, Inosetol, C, D, and E.

Minerals: Multi-mineral complex.

Also: Acidophilus, Cranberry juice, Lecithin, Protein, Propolis, Multi-enzymes, Uratonic, Unsaturated fatty acids, Watermelon, 3-way herb teas, and other Diuretic tablets.

Helpful foods: Red meats, chicken, tuna, fish liver oil, fruit(citrus and other), green leafy vegetables, soybeans, sunflower seeds, sweet potatoes, and wheat bran.

Juices: Blackcherry, carrot, celery, cucumber, pomegranate, and radish juice.

GANGRENE

SPECIFICS: Gangrene is the reduced or stopped blood flow which results in oxygen deprived tissue. It may be caused by frostbite, poor circulation, hardening of the arteries, diabetes, or could be the result of a wound or injury.

(Beneficial Remedies, Treatments, and Nutrients)

Single herbs: Barberry, Black Cohosh, Cayenne, Echinacea, Ginkgo Biloba, Golden Seal, Kelp, and Licorice.

Vitamins: Multi-vitamin plus A, C, and E.

Minerals: Calcium, Magnesium, Potassium, and Zinc.

Also: DMG, Coenzyme Q10, Germanium, and Proteolytic enzymes.

Helpful foods: Apples, bananas, citrus fruits, broccoli, carrots, green and green leafy vegetables, cheese, herring, oysters, fish liver oils, and aloe vera.

GARDNERELLA VAGINALIS
(refer to Vaginitis - page 168)

GAS (Intestinal)

SPECIFICS: A disorder in the small or large intestine usually caused by the fermentation of food in the colon, producing carbon dioxide and hydrogen. Symptoms include abdominal pain, belching, gas, heartburn, nausea, bloating, and vomiting.

(Beneficial Remedies, Treatments, and Nutrients)

HERBAL COMBINATION: (LG).

PHYSIOLOGIC ACTION: Excellent formula for relieving intestinal gas; also cleanses liver and gall bladder.

Single herbs: Catnip, Ginger, Peppermint, and Horseradish are helpful for colon gas.

HOMEOPATHIC COMBINATION: Indigestion & Gas Formula.

Vitamins: B complex, B1, and B5.

Also: Eucarbon, Primadophilus, #8 tissue salts, and activated charcoal.

Helpful foods: Brewers yeast, beets, all seeds and nuts, milk and dairy products, beef, whole grain breads and cereals, and sprouted seeds.

GASTRITIS

SPECIFICS: Gastritis is a disease in which the mucous lining of the stomach becomes inflamed and irritated. Diet and lifestyle influence this condition. It is important to avoid all food irritants such as spices, fried foods, and fiber. Alcohol, aspirin, and coffee irritate the stomach lining. Avoid acidic foods such as tomatoes and citrus fruits. Stress reduction is important in the treatment of gastritis.

(Beneficial Remedies, Treatments, and Nutrients)

Single herbs: Calamus, Chamomile, Dandelion, Marshmallow, Meadowsweet, and Swedish Bitters.

Vitamins: A, B complex, B6, B12, C, D, and E.

Minerals: Calcium, and Iron.

Also: Lecithin, and Linoleic acid.

Helpful foods: Raw vegetables, vegetable oils, fish and fish liver oils, black molasses, yogurt, cheese and other dairy products.

GERMAN MEASLES
(refer to Measles - page 106)

GINGIVITIS

SPECIFICS: Gingivitis is an inflammation of the bones and gums that surround and support the teeth. This disease accounts for the loss of more teeth than cavities, caused by improper cleaning of teeth and gums, poorly fitting dentures, loose fillings, or an inadequate diet.

(Beneficial Remedies, Treatments, and Nutrients)

Single herbs: Chamomile, Echinacea, Lobelia, Myrrh Gum, and White Oak Bark.

Vitamins: A, B complex, C, D, P, Niacin, and Folic Acid.

Minerals: Calcium, Copper, Magnesium, Manganese, Phosphorus, Potassium, Silicon, Sodium, and Zinc.

Also: Coenzyme Q10, Protein, and Unsaturated fatty acids.

Helpful foods: Green leafy vegetables, nuts, oat bran, apples, apricots, bananas, citrus fruits, and seafood.

Juices: Beet greens, celery, green kale, and parsley juice.

GLAND INFECTIONS

SPECIFICS: The lymph glands act as a filter, removing poisons from the blood stream. If the lymph glands are overworked, you will feel run down due to an overload of toxins. A person should cleanse his or her blood at least once every six months.

(Beneficial Remedies, Treatments, and Nutrients)

HERBAL COMBINATION: (IGL).

PHYSIOLOGIC ACTION: Combats infection and reduces inflammation from the body, especially the lymphatic system, ears, throat, lungs, breasts, and organs of the body.

Vitamins: C.

Also: Propolis, Golden Seal, Pau d'Arco, Saw Palmetto, and Echinacea.

Helpful foods: Apples, black currants, cherries, strawberries, citrus fruits, cabbage, green bell peppers, guavas, persimmons, turnip greens, and tomatoes.

Juices: Carrot and Blackberry juice.

GLAND PROBLEMS

SPECIFICS: When the body is under stress, the nutrients in the glands are depleted and the glands, like all body parts, need nutritional replenishment. If one gland malfunctions and is not treated, it puts more stress on all of the other glands. Maintain a well-balanced diet, high in vitamins, minerals and multi glandulars.

(Beneficial Remedies, Treatments, and Nutrients)

HERBAL COMBINATIONS: (GL) (IF).

PHYSIOLOGIC ACTION: Effective for swollen lymph nodes and in helping the body fight glandular weakness and infections.

Single herbs: Alfalfa, Calendula, Echinacea, Golden Seal, Lobelia, Mullein, Saw Palmetto, and Skullcap.

Vitamins: A, B5, B complex, C, and E.

Minerals: Calcium, Magnesium, and Potassium.

Also: Multi Glandulars and Primrose oil.

Helpful foods: Apples, bananas, grapes, citrus fruits, broccoli, carrots, cheese, red meat, fish, chicken, soybeans, sweet potatoes, and turnip greens.

Juices: Carrot, tomato, and pineapple.

GLANDULAR FEVER

SPECIFICS: An infectious disease believed to be caused by a virus. It affects the respiratory system, liver, the lymph tissues, and glands. The disease can be transmitted through communal drinking utensils, kissing, and blood transfusions. A well-balanced diet, adequate in protein, is essential for the prevention of glandular fever.

(Beneficial Remedies, Treatments, and Nutrients)

Single herbs: Dandelion, Echinacea, Goldenseal, Pau d'Arco, and Sheep Sorrel.

Vitamins: A, B complex, B1, B2, B5, B6, C, Biotin, and Choline.

Minerals: Potassium.

Also: Canaid herbal drink, a nondairy form of Acidophilus, Germanium, Raw thymus, Raw glandular complex, and Protein.

Helpful foods: Aloe Vera, bananas, melons, citrus fruits, nuts, oat bran, green leafy vegetables, sweet potatoes, turnip greens, carrots, and fish liver oils.

GLAUCOMA (Hypertension of the eye)

SPECIFICS: Glaucoma is characterized by an increase in pressure of the fluid within the eyeball and a hardening of the surface of the eyeball. The main causes of this disease are related to stress and nutritional problems. It is believed that restoration of vision lost due to nerve degeneration cannot occur. However the vitamins and herbs listed can be effective in controlling and preserving the remaining sight.

(Beneficial Remedies, Treatments, and Nutrients)

HERBAL SUPPLEMENTATION: Eyebright Formula, KB, Bilberry, and Extress.

PHYSIOLOGIC ACTION: These herbs work to restore balance to the system. They supply nutrition to the eye, while helping to remove excessive fluids and toxins. They also help to reduce problems associated with stress.

<u>**Note:**</u> It is important to keep in contact with your doctor while working with this serious eye problem.

HERB COMBINATION: (Eyebright Comb).

Single herbs: Eyebright, Bayberry Bark, Cayenne, Golden Seal, and Red Rasberry.

Vitamins: A, B2, B5, B complex, C, D, and E.

Minerals: A comprehensive multi-mineral formula.

Also: Germanium.

WARNING: Avoid the use of antihistamines, tranquilizers, the herb licorice, and high amounts of niacin.

Helpful foods: Aloe Vera, carrot juice, all fruits, raw vegetables, melon, nuts, seeds, soybeans, sprouted seeds, and sweet potatoes.

GLUTEN ENTEROPATHY

SPECIFICS: Gluten enteropathy is an intestinal disorder caused by the intolerance to a protein in wheat, barley, and rye called gluten. Treatment includes eating a well-balanced gluten-free diet, high in proteins, calories, and normal in fats. Exclude all cereal grains except corn and rice.

(Beneficial Remedies, Treatments, and Nutrients)

Vitamins: A, B6, B12, B complex, C, D, E, and K.

Minerals: Calcium, Iron, Magnesium, and Potassium.

Helpful foods: Apples, bananas, beets, black molasses, carrots, cheese, butter, goats milk, all fruit, kelp, and green leafy vegetables.

GOITER

SPECIFICS: Goiter is the enlargement of the thyroid gland located at the base of the neck. Thyroid disorders are caused by a lack of iodine in the diet, resulting in insufficient thyroxin production or a disorder in the body that requires more thyroxin than the thyroid can produce.

(Beneficial Remedies, Treatments, and Nutrients)

Single herbs: Kelp is an excellent source of iodine.

Vitamins: A, B6, B complex, Choline, C, and E.

Minerals: Calcium and Iodine.

Also: Protein.

Helpful foods: Beef, fish liver oils, dulse and other seaweed, broccoli, carrots, pineapple, citrus fruits, cheese, milk, soybeans, and spinach.

GONORRHEA

SPECIFICS: Gonorrhea is transmitted through sexual intimacy or from the mother to the newborn infant as it passes through the infected birth canal. Complications of gonorrhea may result in sterility in both sexes. Penicillin or another antibiotic is the usual treatment. In addition to medical treatment, an afflicted person should maintain a high nutrient diet to help repair the tissue damage that has occurred.

(Beneficial Remedies, Treatments, and Nutrients)

Single herbs: Echinacea, Goldenseal, Pau d'Arco and Suma.

Vitamins: B complex and K.

Minerals: Zinc.

Also: Acidophilus, Coenzyme Q10, Germanium, and Protein.

Helpful foods: All red meats, fruits, aloe vera, kelp, herring, oysters, liver, nuts, and yogurt.

GOUT

SPECIFICS: This disease occurs when there is an excess of uric acid in the blood and deposits of uric acid salts in the tissue around the joints. Obesity and an improper diet increase an individual's susceptibility to gout. All purine-rich foods need to be avoided, such as anchovies, herring, sardines, mushrooms, mussels, and liver. Treatment requires a low purine diet, generous in vitamins and minerals.

(Beneficial Remedies, Treatments, and Nutrients)

HERBAL COMBINATION: (Yucca AR) (Rheum Aid).

PHYSIOLOGIC ACTION: This formula is effective in helping to reduce swelling and inflammation in body joints and connective tissues. Also helps relieve stiffness and pain.

Single herbs: Burdock, Dandelion Root, Lobelia, Stinging nettle, Safflower, Pau d'Arco, and Yucca.

Vitamins: A, B complex, B5, C, and E.

Minerals: Calcium, Magnesium, and Potassium.

Also: Yu-ccan herbal drink, Primadophilus, Protein, and diet play a vital function in the treatment of this malady. Foods containing Uric Acids, such as meat, and rich pastries need to be avoided.

Helpful foods: Raw vegetables, fish liver oils, dairy products, green leafy vegetables, and whole wheat.

Juices: Celery and parsley juice.

GRIPPE
(refer to Colds and Flu - page 45)

GROWTH PROBLEMS

SPECIFICS: Growth problems occur when there is a malfunction in the thyroid gland or the pituitary gland. The pituitary gland is responsible for the distribution of the growth hormone (somatotropin). An overproduction as well as an underproduction of somatotropin will cause growth abnormalities. Growth problems are also caused by a malfunction of the thyroid gland. Malnutrition plays a significant role in growth and development.

(Beneficial Remedies, Treatments, and Nutrients)

Single herbs: Kelp.

Vitamins: A multi-vitamin plus B complex, and B6.

Minerals: Calcium and Magnesium.

Also: Cod liver oil, L-Lysine, L-Ornithine, Protein, Raw pituitary glandular, and Unsaturated fatty acids.

Helpful foods: Apples, bananas, citrus fruits, cantaloupe, beef, eggs, cheese and other dairy products, kelp, nuts, wheat germ, and wheat bran.

GYNECOLOGICAL PROBLEMS

SPECIFICS: Menstruation is the cyclical process that continuously prepares the uterus for pregnancy, starting at puberty and continuing through menopause.

If this cycle is interrupted or irregular many gynecological problems can occur. Most problems are due to a deficiency of nutrients, this allows infections and viruses to invade the system. (Refer to Premenstrual Syndrome -PMS).

(Beneficial Remedies, Treatments, and Nutrients)

HERBAL COMBINATION: (Fem-Mend).

PHYSIOLOGIC ACTION: Menstrual regulator, tonic for genito-urinary system. Helpful for severe menstrual discomforts. Acts as an aid in rebuilding a malfunctioning reproductive system (Uterus, ovaries, fallopian tubes, etc.).

Single herbs: Aloe Vera, Blessed Thistle, Comfrey Root, Garlic, Ginger, Golden Seal Root, Red Raspberry, Slippery Elm Bark, Uva Ursi, and Yellow Dock Root.

Vitamins: A, B complex, C, and E.

Minerals: A complete multi-mineral.

Helpful foods: Beef, fish and fish liver oils, broccoli, carrots, fruit(citrus and other), green leafy vegetables, liver, nuts, soybeans, and sweet potatoes.

HAIR PROBLEMS

SPECIFICS: Good hygiene and a well-balanced diet is most important for healthy hair. Most hair problems such as balding, graying, dry and brittle hair, etc. can be prevented by nutritional means. There is no known cure to hair loss in males due to heredity. If one is a victim of hair problems due to acute illness, pregnancy, surgery, poor circulation, or stress, the following nutrients can be helpful.

(Beneficial Remedies, Treatments, and Nutrients)

Single herbs: Aloe Vera, Horsetail, Kelp, Rosemary, Sage, Nettle, Yarrow and Yucca.

Vitamins: A, B complex, B3, B5, B6. C, Biotin, Folic Acid, and Inositol.

Minerals: Copper, Iodine, and Magnesium.

Also: Coenzyme Q10, L-Cysteine, L-Methionine, Primadophilus, Protein, Raw thymus glandular, Unsaturated fatty acids, Yu-ccan herbal drink.

Helpful foods: Apples, pineapple, raisins, citrus fruits, dulse and other seaweed, nuts, beef, seafood, turnip greens, broccoli, and carrots.

Juices: Blackcherry juice.

HALITOSIS *(Bad breath)*

SPECIFICS: Halitosis is generally attributed to putrefactive bacteria living on undigested food. Nutrients necessary for efficient digestion are essential. Other causes are poor dental hygiene (gum or tooth decay), nose or throat infection, excessive smoking, liver malfunction, and constipation.

(Beneficial Remedies, Treatments, and Nutrients)

Single herbs: Chlorophyll, Myrrh, Parsley, Peppermint, Rosemary, Sage, and Yucca.

Vitamins: A, B complex, B3, B6, C, and Paba.

Minerals: Magnesium, and Zinc.

Also: Yu-ccan herbal drink, Primadophilus and Digestive enzymes.

Helpful foods: Apples, citrus fruits, green leafy vegetables, turnip greens, yellow corn, nuts, and unpolished rice.

HANGNAILS
(refer to Nail Problems - page 118)

HANGOVER

SPECIFICS: A chronic physiological or psychological condition marked by overindulgence of alcohol. Deficiencies of many nutrients occur when alcohol itself satisfies the body's caloric needs. If the person knows that he or she will be drinking to excess in advance, it is advisable to take vitamin C and a B complex before the party begins. The following vitamins and minerals will also be useful if taken before retiring for the night and the morning after.

(Beneficial Remedies, Treatments, and Nutrients)

Vitamins: A, B complex, B1, B2, B6, B12, Choline, Folic acid, Niacin, Pangamic acid, Pantothenic acid, C, D, E, and K.

Minerals: Calcium, Chromium, Iron, Magnesium, Manganese, Selenium, and Zinc.

HARDENING OF ARTERIES

SPECIFICS: The thickening and hardening of the walls of the arteries is due to the gradual build-up of calcium and fatty deposits on the inside of the artery walls.

This buildup will slow or restrict the circulation of the blood causing high blood pressure. Symptoms of hardening of arteries are cramping of muscles, chest pains and pressure, and hypertension. The main causes are poor diet, drug abuse, alcoholism, smoking, heredity, obesity, and stress.

(Beneficial Remedies, Treatments, and Nutrients)

HERBAL COMBINATION: (Garlicin HC).

PHYSIOLOGIC ACTION: A combination of herbs which supports the cardiovascular system. Helps to strengthen the heart, while building and cleansing the arteries and veins.

Note: Recent animal studies suggest that vitamin C deficiency could be involved in the causation of arteriosclerosis. E.F.A.s (essential fatty acids) play a fundamental role in keeping cell membranes fluid and flexible.

Single herbs: Cayenne, Comfrey, Evening Primrose Oil, Fish Oil, Garlic, Golden Seal, and Rose Hips.

Vitamins: B complex, C, E, Niacin, Inositol, and Choline.

Minerals: Calcium and Magnesium

Also: (E.F.A.s) — Fish oils and cold pressed vegetable oils.

Helpful foods: Fish and fish liver oils, vegetable oils, oat bran, high fiber fruits, kelp, green tea, yogurt, and legumes.

Juices: Alfalfa, beet, blackberry, grape, parsley, and pineapple juice.

HASHIMOTO'S THYROIDITIS
(refer to Hypothyroidism - page 90)

HAY FEVER (Allergic rhinitis)

SPECIFICS: A reaction of the mucous membranes of the nose, eyes, and air passages to animal hair and skin, dust, feathers, pollen, and other irritants. Symptoms include sneezing, itchy eyes, nervous irritability, and a watery discharge from the nose and eyes.

(Beneficial Remedies, Treatments, and Nutrients)

HERBAL COMBINATIONS: (HAS Original and Fast Acting Formulas) (Allergy Care).

PHYSIOLOGIC ACTION: These herbal formulas contain a natural extract of Pseudoepheda, in a base of herbs, which help to restore free breathing without causing drowsiness. HAS original is for those sensitive to Ephedra.

Single herbs: EchinaGuard, Nettle tea, Elder Flowers, Eye Bright, Golden Seal, Golden Rod, Swedish Bitters, and Yarrow

HOMEOPATHIC COMBINATION: Allergy Formula.

Vitamins: A, B complex, B6, Ester C with Bioflavanoids, and E.

Also: Coenzyme Q10, Bee pollen granules or tablets, and Pollen-rich unprocessed raw honey.

Helpful foods: Apple, papaya, broccoli, carrots, green leafy vegetables, soybeans, sweet potatoes, turnip greens, fish and fish liver oils, red meat, and vegetable oils.

Juices: Carrot, celery, and papaya juice.

Note: It is recommended that one reduces consumption of dairy products, white flour products, sugar, and canned foods.

HEADACHE

SPECIFICS: Most common headaches are caused by stress and tension, fevers brought on by allergies or infection, or disturbances of the digestive tract and circulatory system. The following nutrients are beneficial in the treatment the common headache.

(Beneficial Remedies, Treatments, and Nutrients)

Single herbs: Chamomile and Feverfew.

PHYSIOLOGIC ACTION: Chamomile will prevent migraine headaches. Feverfew reduces fever. Feverfew has been historically used for chills and pain that accompany fever. Because of its anecdotal claims for migraine sufferers, it is presently being researched at the London Migraine Clinic.

HOMEOPATHIC COMBINATION: Tension Headache Formula.

Vitamins: A, B1, B2, B3, B6, B12, B complex, C, D, E, and F.

Minerals: Calcium, Iron, Magnesium, Potassium, and Zinc.

Also: Acidophilus and Coenzyme Q10.

Helpful foods: Almonds, apples, avocados, bananas, black molasses, carrots, broccoli, spinach, cheese and other dairy products, herring, and oysters.

HEART ATTACK
(refer to Myocardial Infraction - page 117)

HEART DISEASE

SPECIFICS: The heart is the most important organ of the circulatory
system. If the coronary arteries supplying the heart with blood become plugged or hardened, the flow of oxygen to the heart will be reduced causing severe pain (angina).
Most heart problems are caused by cardiovascular disease. Refer to arteriosclerosis in this manual.

(Beneficial Remedies, Treatments, and Nutrients)

HERBAL COMBINATIONS: (H) (Garlicin HC).

PHYSIOLOGIC ACTION: Promotes elasticity of arteries. Helps eliminate cholesterol; also aids in rebuilding the heart, strengthening and regulating the beat of the heart, and improving circulation in general.

Single herbs: Barberry, Cayenne, Garlic, Hawthorn Berries, Lobelia, and Shepherds Purse.

Vitamins: A, B1, B5, B15, C, D, E, Lecithin, Biotin, Inositol, Choline, and Folic acid.

Minerals: Calcium, Copper, Iodine, Iron, Magnesium, and Potassium.

Helpful foods: Fish and fish liver oils, vegetable oils, oat bran, high fiber fruits, kelp, legumes, green tea, yogurt, and legumes.

Juices: Alfalfa, beet, blackberry, grape, parsley, and pineapple juice.

HEART BURN

SPECIFICS: A burning sensation in the stomach that occurs when hydrochloric acid backs up into the esophagus. Heartburn is caused by allergies, enzyme deficiency, gallbladder problems, hiatal hernia, ulcers, or excessive consumption of spicy and fatty foods.

(Beneficial Remedies, Treatments, and Nutrients)

HERBAL COMBINATION: (Motion Mate).

Single herbs: Chamomile, Chewable Papaya, Meadowsweet, and Marshmallow Root.

Also: Digestive enzymes (especially Pancreatic enzymes), bone meal, and primadophilus.

Helpful foods: Raw fruits and vegetables.

Juices: Carrot, fig, and parsley juice.

HEEL SPUR

SPECIFICS: A painful pointed growth on the bone, most commonly located on the heel. Bone spurs are usually caused by calcium deposits and are common in people who have alkaloses, arthritis, neuritis, and tendonitis.

(Beneficial Remedies, Treatments, and Nutrients)

Vitamins: B6, B complex, and C.

Minerals: Calcium and Magnesium.

Also: Bioflavonoids and Proteolytic enzymes.

Helpful foods: Apples, citrus fruits, sardines, fish liver oils, broccoli, sweet potatoes, turnip greens, unpolished rice, and yellow corn.

HEMOPHILIA

SPECIFICS: A hereditary blood disease that is found only in men. The blood of hemophiliacs fails to clot or coagulation as time is prolonged. Transfusion of fresh whole blood or plasma is required to provide necessary coagulation in emergencies.

(Beneficial Remedies, Treatments, and Nutrients)

Single herbs: Barley Grass, Beet Powder, Black Current, Chlorophyll, Chlorella, Comfrey, Dandelion, Fenugreek, Kelp, and Yellowdock.

Vitamins: A multi-vitamin and additional C and E.

Minerals: Complete multi-mineral.

Also: Desiccated liver.

Helpful foods: Red meats, liver, citrus fruits, vegetable oils, and whole wheat.

HEMORRHOIDS

SPECIFICS: Hemorrhoids are swollen or ruptured veins located around the anus that may protrude out of the rectum. The most common cause is strain on the abdominal muscles due to constipation, improper lifting, and pregnancy. Prevention and treatment include an improved diet containing fluids and fiber and exercise.

(Beneficial Remedies, Treatments, and Nutrients)

HERBAL COMBINATION: (Yellow Dock Formula).

PHYSIOLOGIC ACTION: Effective formula for hemorrhoids, colitis, and blood purifier. Also revitalizes prolapsed uterus, kidneys, and bowl.

Single herbs: Butchers Broom, Collinsonia Root, Horse chestnut, Lobelia, Stone Root, and Yellow Dock.

HOMEOPATHIC COMBINATION: Constipation and Hemorrhoids Formula.

Vitamins: A, B complex, Choline, Inositol, B6, C, E, and P.

Minerals: Multi-mineral complex plus Calcium.

Also: Coenzyme Q10, Bulk forming laxatives such as Laxacil, or Psyllium seed husks are recommended to take pressure from the colon. Combination "Hem Relief" ointment, Pile ointment and suppositories, or Circu Caps Witch Hazel Compresses.

Helpful foods: Apricots, cherries, grapes, citrus fruits, broccoli, carrots, green leafy vegetables, oats, soybeans, beef, fish, and whole wheat bread.

Juices: Celery, grapefruit, and spinach juice.

HEPATITIS

SPECIFICS: An inflammation of the liver caused by infection or toxic agents. The liver is unable to eliminate poisons and it cannot store and process certain nutrients that are vital for the body. Recovery from hepatitis requires a diet adequate in all nutrients, abstention from alcohol, and rest.
Sensitivity to toxic materials may persist so B complex, C, and E should be continued long after recovery.

(Beneficial Remedies, Treatments, and Nutrients)

Single herbs: Dandelion, Goldenseal, Milk Thistle, and Red Clover.

Vitamins: A, B complex, B6, Pangamic acid, Pantothenic acid, C, and E.

Minerals: Zinc.

Also: Coenzyme Q10, Fluids, Germanium, Lecithin, Multienzymes, Protein, Raw liver extract, and Unsaturated fatty acids.

Helpful foods: Aloe Vera, broccoli, carrots, spinach, turnip greens, soybeans, sweet potatoes, garlic, herring, oysters, fish liver oils, and vegetable oils.

Juices: Grapefruit, sauerkraut, and tomato juice.

HERPES SIMPLEX (I and II)

SPECIFICS: Herpes simplex 1 results in cold sores and skin eruptions. It can also cause inflammation of the eye. If the eye becomes infected see a doctor at once. Herpes simplex 2 is sexually transmitted and results in lesions on the penis in men and infection inside the vagina in women. After entering the body the herpes virus never leaves. By strengthening the immune system one can defend against or prevent herpes activation.

(Beneficial Remedies, Treatments, and Nutrients)

Single herbs: Echinacea, Goldenseal, Myrrh, Red Clover, and Turkish Rhubarb.

Vitamins: B complex, C, and E.

Minerals: Zinc chelate.

Also: Canaid herbal drink strengthens the immune system and the amino acid L-Lysine has a direct effect on the virus.

Helpful foods: Raw vegetables, all fruits and melons, vegetable oils, soybeans, and whole grains.

HIATAL HERNIA

SPECIFICS: Over fifty percent of the population, over the age of forty, experience hiatal hernia. This condition is caused by a hole in the diaphragm muscles. Heartburn and ulcers can occur due to the leakage of stomach acid back into the lower esophagus.
 The victim suffers from discomfort behind the breastbone, heartburn, and a burning sensation in the throat caused by the acid coming up into the throat.

(Beneficial Remedies, Treatments, and Nutrients)

Single herbs: Aloe Vera juice, Comfrey, Goldenseal, and Red Clover.

Vitamins: Multi-vitamin plus A, B complex, B12, and C.

Minerals: Multi-mineral plus Zinc.

Also: Pancreatin, Papaya, and Proteolytic enzymes.

Helpful foods: Beef, broccoli, carrots, green leafy vegetables, all fruit, melon, nuts, herring, oysters, fish liver oils, and unpolished rice.

HOOKWORMS

SPECIFICS: Hookworms live in the gastrointestinal tract. Early signs include diarrhea, loss of appetite, and rectal itching. If not eliminated they will result in the loss of weight, colon disorders,
and anemia. Causes include ingestion of eggs or larvae from partially cooked meat, improper disposal of human waste, and walking barefoot on contaminated soil.

(Beneficial Remedies, Treatments, and Nutrients)

HERBAL COMBINATIONS: (Para-X) (Para-VF).

PHYSIOLOGIC ACTION: Useful in destroying and eliminating parasites, such as worms. Also helps relieve many kinds of skin problems. The Para-VF is liquid and is useful for children and the elderly, who cannot swallow capsules.

WARNING: Do not use during pregnancy!

Single herbs: Black Walnut, Garlic, Pumpkin Seeds, Sage, Sheep Sorrel, Swedish Bitters, and Wormwood.

Vitamins: Folic Acid.

Children: Chamomile tea or raisins soaked in Senna tea, for older children, may be helpful.

Helpful foods: Asparagus, brewers yeast, lettuce, liver, mushrooms, nuts, lima beans, and wheat germ.

HORMONE REGULATION

SPECIFICS: A hormonal imbalance is always experienced at the point at which women stop ovulating, the end of their reproductive years, or during puberty. Symptoms include difficult breathing, dizziness, headache, heart palpitations, hot flashes, and depression. The following nutrients will help regulate the hormones and alleviate the symptoms in both cases.

(Beneficial Remedies, Treatments, and Nutrients)

FEMALE HERBAL COMBINATIONS: (MP) or (Change-O-Life).

PHYSIOLOGIC ACTION: This herbal formula is effective in regulating hormonal imbalance. Its greatest benefit is for the relief of the symptoms of menopause. Also good for youth during puberty.

Single herbs: Blessed Thistle, Damiana, Dong Quai, Mistletoe, and Vitex Agnus Castus.

HOMEOPATHIC COMBINATION: Menopause Formula.

MALE HERB COMBINATION: (APH).

PHYSIOLOGIC ACTION: Stimulates sexual impulses and strengthens and increases sexual power. Helps eliminate fatigue and increases longevity.

Single herbs: Damiana, Fo-Ti, Gota Kola, Sarsaparilla Root, Saw Palmetto, and Siberian Ginseng.

Minerals: Potassium.

Helpful foods: All vegetables, bananas, cantaloupe, citrus fruits, milk, mint leaves, potatoes, sunflower seeds, tomatoes, watercress, and whole wheat.

HORMONE IMBALANCE
(Refer to Menopause)

HOT FLASHES
(refer to Menopause - page 109)

HOUSEMAID'S KNEE

SPECIFICS: Housemaid's knee is an inflammation of the bursae, liquid filled sacs found in the joints, tendons, muscles, and bones. This disorder is caused by prolonged kneeling on a hard surface, causing swelling, tenderness, and extreme pain. During infection, elevated doses of A, C, and E are beneficial in the treatment of bursitis.

(Beneficial Remedies, Treatments, and Nutrients)

HERBAL COMBINATIONS: (Rheum-Aid) (Cal-Silica) (Kalmin).

PHYSIOLOGIC ACTIONS: These herbal combinations contain herbs which exhibit anti-inflammatory and relaxing effects. Help to build nerve tissue and relieve stiffness and pain.

Single herbs: Alfalfa, Chaparral, and Comfrey. Mullein is often used as a poultice to give relief externally.

Vitamins: A, B12, B complex, C, E, and P.

Minerals: Calcium and Magnesium.

Also: Alkaline diet, Coenzyme Q10, Germanium, Proteolytic enzymes, and a protein supplement.

Helpful foods: Apples, apricots, cherries, citrus fruits, sardines, tuna, fish liver oils, spinach, and sweet potatoes.

HYPERACTIVITY

SPECIFICS: A disorder of certain mechanisms in the central nervous system. This disorder is usually caused by a diet high in refined carbohydrates, a result of boredom, or feelings of insecurity.

(Beneficial Remedies, Treatments, and Nutrients)

HERBAL COMBINATION: (Wild Lettuce and Valerian Extract).

PHYSIOLOGIC ACTION: This excellent formula is a natural sedative. Promotes overall calming of the nerves and restores a sense of control and balance without causing drowsiness.

Also: Ginkgo or Ginkgold. Although this herb is often used to promote circulation, it also has a positive effect on the nervous system. Used in conjunction with the following single herbs and with a balanced, chemical free diet, good results can be expected.

Single herbs: Evening Primrose Oil, Lobelia, Oat Extract, Skullcap, St. John's Wort, Valerian, Wild Lettuce, and Yucca.

Vitamins: High potency B vitamins, B3, B5, B6, and C.

Note: Yeast free B vitamins may be required if yeast intolerance is present.

Minerals: High doses of all minerals.

Helpful foods: Red meats, chicken, green leafy vegetables, nuts, turnip greens, and unpolished rice.

Note: Avoid all foods with artificial flavoring and coloring. Processed foods should be eliminated from the diet. Foods which contain natural salicylates such as apples, tomatoes, and oranges need to be avoided. Carbonated drinks will worsen the condition.

HYPERTENTION

SPECIFICS: The main cause of hypertention is arteriosclerosis. This condition is due to the gradual build-up of calcium and fatty deposits on the inside of the artery walls. This buildup will slow or restrict the circulation of the blood causing high blood pressure. Symptoms of high blood pressure are cramping of muscles, chest pains and pressure, and hypertension. Causes for high blood pressure are poor diet, drug abuse, alcoholism, smoking, heredity, obesity, and stress.

(Beneficial Remedies, Treatments, and Nutrients)

HERBAL COMBINATIONS: (Cayenne-Garlic) (Garlicin HC) (BP)

PHYSIOLOGIC ACTION: In addition to lowering the blood pressure, the above will help to relieve colds, influenza, and general infections, strengthen the heart and improves blood circulation.

Single herbs: Cayenne, Garlic, Kelp, Hawthorn, Mistletoe, Valerian Root, Yarrow, and Yucca.

Vitamins: A, B complex (stress) B3, B5, B15, C, D, E, P, Inositol, Choline, and Lecithin

Minerals: Calcium, Magnesium, and Potassium.

Helpful foods: Apples, apricots, bananas, cherries, broccoli, carrots, green leafy vegetables, soybeans, sunflower seeds, vegetable oils, and fish liver oils.

Juices: Carrot, celery, grape, and lime juice.

HYPERTHYROIDISM

SPECIFICS: When the body is under stress, the nutrients in the glands are depleted and the glands, like all body parts, need nutritional replenishment. If one gland malfunctions and is not treated, it puts more stress on all of the other glands. Maintain a well-balanced diet, high in vitamins, minerals and multi glandulars.

(Beneficial Remedies, Treatments, and Nutrients)

HERBAL COMBINATIONS: (GL) (IF).

PHYSIOLOGIC ACTION: Effective for swollen lymph nodes and in helping the body fight glandular weakness and infections.

Single herbs: Alfalfa, Calendula, Echinacea, Golden Seal, Lobelia, Mullein, Saw Palmetto, and Skullcap.

Vitamins: A, B5, B complex, C, and E.

Minerals: Calcium, Magnesium, and Potassium.

Also: Multi Glandulars and Primrose oil.

Helpful foods: Apples, bananas, grapes, citrus fruits, broccoli, carrots, cheese, red meat, fish, chicken, soybeans, sweet potatoes, and turnip greens.

Juices: Carrot, tomato, and pineapple.

HYPOCALCEMIA
(refer to Calcium Deficiency - page 33)

HYPOGLYCEMIA

SPECIFICS: Hypoglycemia is caused by the over secretion of insulin by the pancreas, resulting in an abnormally low level of glucose or sugar in the blood. Hypoglycemia can contribute to allergies, arthritis, asthma, epilepsy, impotence, and mental disorders. A proper diet is the main factor in maintaining proper blood sugar levels.

(Beneficial Remedies, Treatments, and Nutrients)

HERBAL COMBINATIONS: (HIGL) (AdrenAid).

PHYSIOLOGIC ACTION: Stimulates the adrenals and the pancreas to help restore sugar levels, helps correct glandular imbal-ances, eliminates toxins, assists the body in handling stressful conditions, and promotes a feeling of well-being.

WARNING: Some people who have hypoglycemia cannot handle Golden Seal, as it tends to lower the blood sugar level. Safflower is good to take before exercise.

Vitamins: A, B1, B2, B3, B6, B9, B12, B complex, C, and E.

Minerals: Magnesium and Potassium.

Also: Bee Pollen, Juniper, Glyco-lite, Acidophilus. Low animal protein, small meals high in natural complex carbohydrates.

Helpful foods: All vegetables, apples, apricots, bananas, citrus fruits, oat bran, vegetable oils, and whole wheat bread.

HYPOTENTION
(refer to Blood Pressure Low - page 25)

HYPOTHYROIDISM

SPECIFICS: A disorder that occurs when there is an underproduction of hormones by the thyroid gland, resulting in lowered cellular metabolism. In this disorder, the brain cells are effected and intellectual capacity is impaired. Problems with the thyroid gland can be the cause of many recurring illnesses, infections, and chronic fatigue.

(Beneficial Remedies, Treatments, and Nutrients)

HERBAL COMBINATION: (T).

PHYSIOLOGIC ACTION: Rich in natural vitamins and minerals, this excellent formula helps revitalize and promote healing of the thyroid glands, thus restoring metabolism balance. Helps the body store up needed vitality and energy.

Single herbs: Black Walnut, Irish Moss, Kelp, Mullein, and Parsley.

Vitamins: B1, B5, C, D, E, and F.

Minerals: Chlorine, Iodine, Potassium, and Zinc.

Also: Brewer's yeast, Essential fatty acids, Lecithin, Protein, and Thyroid glandular.

Helpful foods: Broccoli, carrots, green leafy vegetables, soybeans, turnip greens, sweet potatoes, vegetable oils, fish liver oils, citrus fruits, and melons.

Juices: Celery and clam juice.

ICTERUS
(refer to Jaundice - page 95)

ILEITIS
(refer to Crohn's Disease - page 51)

IMPETIGO

SPECIFICS: This condition is best looked after with a good blood cleanser and a vitamin and mineral rich diet.

(Beneficial Remedies, Treatments, and Nutrients)

HERBAL COMBINATIONS: (Red Clover Combination) (Yellow Dock Formula) (AKN).

PHYSIOLOGIC ACTION: These herbal formulas effectively aid the body's cleansing systems, thus helps eliminate ulcers of the skin, impetigo, etc.

Single herbs: Echinacea, Licorice Root, and Red Clover.

Vitamins: A, C, D, E. Vitamin A and E applied topically. Vitamin A is necessary for the health of the skin tissue and vitamins C, D, and E, may be helpful in aiding the skin in its recovery from impetigo.

Helpful foods: Citrus fruits, fish liver oils, and vegetable oils.

IMMUNE DEFICIENCY

SPECIFICS: When the immune system weakens, you become more susceptible to infections and viruses. The key factors in the treatment and prevention of immune deficiency are proper nutrition and good supplementation.

(Beneficial Remedies, Treatments, and Nutrients)

HERBAL COMBINATION: (EchinaGuard).

PHYSIOLOGIC ACTION: Stimulates the immune response systems. Especially helpful in rebuilding the body during convalescence and as a preventative.

Single herbs: Echinacea root, Chaparral, Korean White Ginseng, Goldenseal root, Pau d'Arco, and Rosemary.

Vitamins: A multi-vitamin plus B6, B12, C, and E.

Minerals: A strong mineral complex.

Also: Canaid herbal drink strengthens the immune system. L-Cysteine, L-Methionine, L-Lysine, L-Ornithine, Propolis, Proteolytic enzymes, and Primadophilus.

Helpful foods: Beef, broccoli, fruit(citrus and other), nuts, soybeans, spinach, sweet potatoes, turnip greens, unpolished rice, and whole grains.

IMPOTENCE

SPECIFICS: The inability to achieve or maintain an erection. Impotence may be psychological or organic in nature. A balanced diet is important. Do not consume animal fats, fried foods, junk foods, or sugar!

(Beneficial Remedies, Treatments, and Nutrients)

HERBAL COMBINATION: (APH).

PHYSIOLOGIC ACTION: Stimulates male and female sexual impulses as well as strengthens and increases sexual power and helps fight fatigue.

Single herbs: Damiana, Ginkgo, Ginseng and Gotu Kola.

Vitamins: E, Paba, Folic acid, and Lecithin.

Minerals: Zinc, Iodine, and Calcium.

Also: L-Arginine, L-Tyrosine, Proteolytic enzymes, Melbrosia (for men), Tropical Impulse tea, Loving Mood, Bee pollen, Sesame seeds, and Ginseng.

Helpful foods: High quality vegetable oil, fertile eggs, raw milk.

Juices: Celery and parsley juice.

INDIGESTION
(refer to Digestive Disorders - page 56)

INFERTILITY

SPECIFICS: The inability to become pregnant or the inability to carry a pregnancy full-term. The following supplements are essential to correcting hormonal imbalance. Because there are so many causes of infertility, it is recommended that you get a qualified doctors opinion.

(Beneficial Remedies, Treatments, and Nutrients)

Single herbs: Dong Quai, and Gotu Kola.

Vitamins: A, B6, B complex, and E.

Minerals: A complete mineral complex.

Also: Astrelin, Gerovital H-3, L-Tyrosine, Proteolytic enzymes, and Raw ovarian concentrate.

Helpful foods: Beef, chicken, fish and fish liver oils, fruit, melons, nuts, soybeans, vegetable oils, green leafy vegetables, and whole grain vegetables.

INFLUENZA
(refer to Colds and Flu - page 45)

INSOMNIA

SPECIFICS: Insomnia is classified as habitual sleeplessness, repeated night after night. Some of the causes of insomnia are asthma, depression, compulsive personality or schizophrenic tendencies, and deficiencies of vitamins, minerals, and enzymes.

(Beneficial Remedies, Treatments, and Nutrients)

HERBAL COMBINATIONS: (E-Z Sleep) (Silent Night).

PHYSIOLOGIC ACTION: Soothing mild relaxant. Promotes natural restful and refreshing sleep.

Single herbs: Catnip, Hops, Lady Slipper, Skullcap, Passionflower, Pau d'Arco, and Valerian root.

HOMEOPATHIC COMBINATION: Insomnia Formula.

Vitamins: B1, B3, B5, B6, D, and E.

Minerals: Calcium, Iron, Magnesium, and Potassium.

Also: Protein and Tryptophan.

Helpful foods: Apples, apricots, bananas, citrus fruits, sprouted seeds, sunflower seeds, whole rye and wheat, and yellow corn.

Juices: Celery and lettuce juice.

INTESTINAL PARASITES

SPECIFICS: There are several types of parasites that can live in human intestines. The most common parasites are hookworms, pinworms, roundworms, and tapeworms. Worms irritate the intestinal lining causing poor absorption of vital nutrients.

(Beneficial Remedies, Treatments, and Nutrients)

HERBAL COMBINATIONS: (Para-X) (Para-VF).

PHYSIOLOGIC ACTION: Useful in destroying and eliminating parasites, such as worms. The Para-VF is liquid and is useful for children and the elderly who cannot swallow capsules.

WARNING: Do not use during pregnancy!

Single herbs: Black Walnut, Garlic, Pumpkin Seeds, Sage, Sheep Sorrel, Swedish Bitters, and Wormwood.

Vitamins: A, B1, B2, B6, B12, B complex, D, and K.

Minerals: Calcium and Iron.

CHILDREN: Chamomile tea or raisins soaked in Senna tea, for older children, may be helpful.

Helpful foods: Raw vegetables and fruits, vegetable oils, and fish liver oils.

IRRITABLE BLADDER
(refer to Kidney and Bladder - page 96)

IRRITABLE BOWEL SYNDROME

SPECIFICS: A common gastrointestinal disorder caused by irregular and uncoordinated muscular contractions of the intestine. This interferes with the movement of waste through the bowels causing the formation of excess toxins and mucus in the bloodstream and bowels.

(Beneficial Remedies, Treatments, and Nutrients)

HERBAL COMBINATION: (Multilax #1) or (Naturalax #1).

PHYSIOLOGIC ACTION: Helps relieve minor constipation.

WARNING: Do not use when abdominal pain nausea or vomiting are present! Frequent or prolonged use of preparation may result in dependence on laxatives.

Also: Yu-ccan herbal drink, Vita Cleansing Tea, Swiss Kriss, Metab Herb, Psyllium Husks, Flax meal, Super D Tea. Drink lots of pure water to flush system.

Helpful foods: Citrus fruits and bananas.

JAUNDICE (NON INFECTIOUS)

SPECIFICS: Jaundice is not in itself a disease, but a sign of a liver, kidney, or blood disorder, which causes a build-up of bilirubin in the blood. Bilirubin is the presence of pigments from worn out blood cells that are deposited in the tissues, causing the skin and whites of the eyes to become abnormally yellow, rather than being excreted in bile as waste products.

(Beneficial Remedies, Treatments, and Nutrients)

HERBAL COMBINATION: (LG).

PHYSIOLOGIC ACTION: This herbal combination helps to correct malfunctioning of the liver and gall bladder. It is a liver detoxifier, and a bile stimulant.

Single herbs: Birch Leaves, Dandelion, Fennel, Horse Tail, Irish Moss, Parsley, and Rose Hips.

Vitamins: A, B6, C, D, and E.

Minerals: Calcium, Magnesium, and Phosphorus.

Also: Lecithin, Protein, and Unsaturated fatty acids.

Helpful foods: Apples, bananas, broccoli, carrots, cheese and other dairy products, tuna, fish liver oils, red meat, vegetable oils, and sprouted seeds.

Juices: Sauerkraut and tomato juice.

JET LAG

SPECIFICS: Siberian ginseng, taken on a regular basis for about a week before the trip, seems to have a balancing effect on the system, lessening the effects of Jet Lag. A good vitamin supplement is also helpful.

(Beneficial Remedies, Treatments, and Nutrients)

Single herbs: Gota Kola and Korean Ginseng.

Vitamins: Stress B Complex, Multi-Vitamin, C, and E.

Minerals: Multi-mineral complex.

Helpful foods: All fruits, spinach, sweet potatoes, turnip greens, and unpolished rice.

KIDNEY AND BLADDER DISORDERS

SPECIFICS: There are many problems that may occur in the kidneys and bladder, however most of the problems are caused by infection. The symptoms of urinary tract infections are loss of appetite, chills, fever, frequency of urination, back pain, nausea, and vomiting.

(Beneficial Remedies, Treatments, and Nutrients)

HERBAL COMBINATION: (KB).

PHYSIOLOGIC ACTION: Extremely valuable in healing and strengthening the kidneys, bladder, and genito-urinary area. Useful to stop bed-wetting, but is a diuretic when congestion of the kidneys is indicated. Helps remove bladder, uterine, and urethral toxins.

WARNING: Intended for occasional use only. May cause green-yellow discoloration of urine.

Single herbs: Alfalfa, Barberry root, Catnip, Dandelion, Fennel, Ginger root, Goldenrod, Horsetail, Uva Ursi, and Wild Yam.

Vitamins: A, B complex, C, D, E, and Choline.

Minerals: Calcium, Magnesium, and Potassium.

Also: Digestive enzymes, Lecithin, L-Arginine, L-Methionine, Propolis, Uratonic, Watermelon, 3-way herb teas, and other Diuretic tablets.

Helpful foods: All vegetables, apples, bananas, broccoli, carrots, cheese and other dairy products, tuna, and fish liver oils, red meat, and sprouted seeds.

Juices: Asparagus, black currant, cranberry, celery, juniper berry, parsley, and pomegranate juice.

KIDNEY FUNCTIONS

SPECIFICS: The kidney is essential to the regulation of the body's acid base balance and fluid balance. Kidney failure is the inability of the kidneys to filter waste products from the blood and excrete them in the urine, to regulate the blood pressure, and to control the body's water and salt balance.

(Beneficial Remedies, Treatments, and Nutrients)

HERBAL COMBINATION: Garlic and Parsley.

PHYSIOLOGIC ACTION: Promotes urine flow and strengthens kidneys. Also revitalizes and strengthens liver and spleen.

Also: Propolis, cranberry juice, 3-way herb teas, and uratonic.

Helpful foods: Refer to Kidney and Bladder in this manual.

KIDNEY AND BLADDER STONES

SPECIFICS: Kidney and bladder stones are abnormal accumulations of mineral salts, combined mostly with calcium, which form in the kidney, but can lodge anywhere along the course of the urinary tract. Symptoms include increased urination that may contain blood or pus, chills, fever, and pain radiating from the upper back to the lower abdomen.

(Beneficial Remedies, Treatments, and Nutrients)

HERBAL COMBINATION: (PR).

PHYSIOLOGIC ACTION: PR combination helps dissolve kidney stones. PR helps keep kidneys flushed out (toxins and buildup of waste and sediments). Juniper keeps kidneys flushed out. Parsley acts as a diuretic. Magnesium helps prevent stones from forming. Thyme helps prevent buildup and dissolves stones if already present.

Single herbs: Corn silk, Dandelion, Ginkgo Biloba extract, Goldenrod, Juniper, Parsley, Sheep Sorrel, Thyme, and Uva Ursi.

Vitamins: A, B2, B5, B6, C, E, F, and Choline.

Minerals: Magnesium and Potassium.

Also: Canaid herbal drink and Proteolytic enzymes.

Helpful foods: All vegetable oils, apples, bananas, broccoli, carrots, cheese and other dairy products, tuna, fish liver oils, red meat, sprouted seeds, unpolished rice, and whole wheat.

Juices: Apple, beet root, lemon, and radish juice.

LABOR AND DELIVERY

SPECIFICS: The process by which an infant moves from the uterus to the outside world. The first stage of labor covers the period from the onset until the woman's cervix is fully dilated. The second stage lasts from full dilatation of the cervix until the birth of the baby. The third stage lasts from the delivery until the afterbirth is expelled.

(Beneficial Remedies, Treatments, and Nutrients)

Single herbs: Red Raspberry.

SPECIFICS: Red Raspberry is essential during labor. It coordinates the uterine contractions often making labor shorter.

LACTOSE INTOLERANCE

SPECIFICS: The inability to properly digest milk and milk products due to a shortage of the enzyme called lactase in the system. Symptoms range from mild abdominal discomfort to bloating, diarrhea, flatulence, and stomachache.

(Beneficial Remedies, Treatments, and Nutrients)

Vitamins: A complete multi-vitamin.

Minerals: Calcium.

Helpful foods: Broccoli, tofo, kale, salmon, and sardines.

LEAD POISONING

SPECIFICS: Lead is one of the most widely used and one of the most toxic metal contaminants in the world today.

A cumulative poison that is retained in bones, brain, central nervous system, and glands. Victims of lead poisoning experience hyperactivity, severe gastrointestinal colic, their gums turn blue, and muscle weakness. Lead poisoning can eventually lead to blindness, loss of memory, mental retardation, and paralysis of the limbs. If you suspect lead poisoning you should drink distilled water and make sure that your diet is high in fiber, supplemented with pectin.

(Beneficial Remedies, Treatments, and Nutrients)

Single herbs: Alfalfa and Kelp.

Vitamins: A, B1, B6, B complex, C, and E.

Minerals: Chromium, Iron, Selenium, and Zinc.

Also: Lecithin, L-Cysteine, L-Cystine, L-Glutathionine, L-Lysine, and L-Methionine.

Helpful foods: Beef, black molasses, oat bran, chicken, herring and oysters, shellfish, mushrooms, fruit(citrus and other), whole rye, and whole wheat.

LEG CRAMPS

SPECIFICS: An involuntary spasm or contraction of the muscle in the leg. Most cramps occur at night after a day of unusual exertion, when the limbs are cool. Leg cramps are caused by impaired blood circulation or a nutritional deficiency.

(Beneficial Remedies, Treatments, and Nutrients)

HERBAL COMBINATION: (Ca-T).

PHYSIOLOGIC ACTION: Effectively calms nerves and aids sleep, in addition to rebuilding the nerve sheath, veins, and artery walls.

Single herbs: Comfrey Herb, Horsetail Grass, Oat Straw, and Skullcap.

Vitamins: B complex, B1, B2, B5, C, D, and E.

Minerals: Calcium, Magnesium, and Phosphorus.

Also: #12 tissue salts, Protein, and Unsaturated fatty acids.

Helpful foods: Red meat, butter, cheese, citrus fruits, soybeans, rice, sunflower seeds, nuts, whole grains, and sweet potatoes.

LEG ULCERS

SPECIFICS: Leg ulcers are caused by poor circulation of blood to the legs. Restricted blood flow causes open sores to develop on deteriorated patches of skin.

(Beneficial Remedies, Treatments, and Nutrients)

HERBAL COMBINATIONS: (H Formula) (Ginkgold).

PHYSIOLOGIC ACTION: Contains herbs which strengthen the heart and builds the vascular system. When taken with Cayenne, it improves circulation, giving a warming sensation to the entire body.

Single herbs: Cayenne, Bayberry, Butchers Broom, Ginkgo, and Yarrow.

Vitamins: A, B3, B12, C, and E.

Minerals: Calcium, Iron, Magnesium, and Potassium.

Also: Coenzyme Q10, Germanium, Lecithin, and Protein.

Helpful foods: Aloe Vera juice, apples, apricots, bananas, all vegetables, citrus fruit, cheese, fish, and beef.

LEGIONNAIRES' DISEASE

SPECIFICS: A lung and bronchial tube infection caused by the bacterial infection called (legionella pneumophilia). At this time modern science knows very little about this disease. It is believed that the bacteria are transmitted through the air, the bacteria which is found at excavation sites, or in newly plowed soil could be transmitted through the skin.

(Beneficial Remedies, Treatments, and Nutrients)

Single herbs: Pau d'Arco, plus Catnip, Echinacea, Eucalyptus, Garlic, and Goldenseal.

Vitamins: A strong multi-vitamin plus A, B complex, and C.

Minerals: Multi-mineral complex plus Zinc.

Also: L-Carnitine, L-Cystine, and Raw thumus.

Helpful foods: Apples, apricots, cherries, citrus fruits, melons, lean beef, broccoli, carrots, green leafy vegetables, nuts, sweet potatoes, turnip greens, and unpolished rice.

LEUKEMIA

SPECIFICS: Leukemia is a fatal blood disease caused by an overproduction of white blood cells.

Acute leukemia is marked by a sudden onset of symptoms and usually occurs in children and young adults. Chronic leukemia is found only in adults and the symptoms develop slower. A well-balanced diet containing all vitamins and minerals will help maintain strength and may possibly extend their lifetime.

(Beneficial Remedies, Treatments, and Nutrients)

Single herbs: Pau d'Arco, Swedish Bitters, and Nettle.

Vitamins: B complex, B12, C, and E.

Minerals: Copper, Iron, and Zinc.

Also: Canaid herbal drink.

Helpful foods: Aloe Vera, apples, bananas, broccoli, oat bran, carrots, citrus fruits, green leafy vegetables, soybeans, sweet potatoes, turnip greens, vegetable oils, lean red meat, and fish liver oils.

Refer to "Cancer".

LEUKORRHEA

SPECIFICS: Leukorrhea is a white vaginal discharge often caused by a one celled microorganism called Trichomonas vaginalis, or by a yeast fungus called monilia.

(Beneficial Remedies, Treatments, and Nutrients)

HERBAL COMBINATION: (Cantrol).

PHYSIOLOGIC ACTION: An excellent well-balanced formula of herbs and supplements which balance the system while killing yeast. It includes caprylic acid and anti-oxidants for the control and eventual elimination of yeast fungus.

Single herbs: Black Walnut, Caprinex, Garlicin, Pau d'Arco, and Yucca.

Note: Drink three cups of Pau d'Arco tea daily. This herb is a natural antibiotic agent.

Vitamins: A, B complex, Biotin, D, and E.

Minerals: Calcium and Magnesium.

Also: Yu-ccan herbal drink, Linseed Oil, Candida Cleanse, Caprilic Acid, and Primadophilus.

Helpful foods: Egg yolk, apricot, citrus fruits, beef kidney, beef liver, vegetable and fish oils.

LIVER and GALLBLADDER DISORDERS

SPECIFICS: The liver is the largest organ of the body and is located under the diaphragm just above the stomach. It is responsible for detoxifying harmful substances such as alcohol, food additives, pesticides, and environmental pollutants. The liver also produces cholesterol, enzymes, lecithin, and bile. The following nutrients are beneficial in the treatment of liver and gallbladder disorders.

(Beneficial Remedies, Treatments, and Nutrients)

HERBAL COMBINATION: (LG).

PHYSIOLOGIC ACTION: Helps the cleansing of the liver and gall bladder; restores new energy to these organs. Also can be taken to relieve intestinal gas.

Single herbs: Bayberry Root, Catnip, Fennel Seed, Ginger Root, and Peppermint.

Vitamins: A, B1, B2, B6, Choline, Niacin, Pantothenic acid, C, and E.

Minerals: Copper and Sulfur for the Liver. Magnesium and Sulfur for the Gallbladder.

Also: Acidophilus, Calamus Root tea, Chlorophyll, Digestive enzymes, and Hydrochloric acid.

Helpful foods: All vegetables, apples, bananas, broccoli, carrots, cheese and other dairy products, tuna and fish liver oils, red meat, and sprouted seeds.

Juices: Beet root, blackcherry, carrot, cucumber, pineapple, and radish juice.

LIVER DISORDERS

SPECIFICS: Refer to liver and gallbladder disorders.

(Beneficial Remedies, Treatments, and Nutrients)

HERBAL COMBINATIONS: (Thisilyn) (Milk Thistle Extract).

PHYSIOLOGIC ACTION: Protects liver. Anti-oxidant quality prevents free radical damage in the liver.

Single herbs: Dandelion and Horsetail.

Vitamins: A, B Complex, B1, B2, B3, B6, Choline, C, and E.

Also: Digestive Enzymes, Lecithin, and Primadophilus.

Helpful foods: Apples, bananas, broccoli, carrots, cheese and other dairy products, tuna and fish liver oils, red meat, vegetable oils, and sprouted seeds.

Juices: Sauerkraut and tomato juice.

LOWER BOWEL PROBLEMS

SPECIFICS: Constipation results when the waste material moves too slowly or there is decreased frequency of bowel movements. Constipation usually arises from insufficient amounts of fiber and fluids in the diet. Other causes include lack of exercise, nervousness, stress, infections, and poor diet.

(Beneficial Remedies, Treatments, and Nutrients)

HERBAL COMBINATIONS: (Multilax #2) or (Naturalax #2)

PHYSIOLOGIC ACTION: Accelerates natural cleansing of the body and improves intestinal absorption by gentle evacuation of bowels. Cleans out old toxic fecal matter, mucus and encrustation's from the colon wall, and helps normalize the peristaltic action and rebuild the bowel structure. Use until the bowel is cleansed, healed, and functioning normally.

Single herbs: Cascara Sagrada, Golden Seal Root, Lobelia, Red Raspberry, Senna, and Yucca.

Vitamins: A multi-vitamin plus the B complex.

Minerals: A strong multi-mineral complex.

Also: Yu-ccan herbal drink, Flax seeds, Psyllium seeds, Whey powder, Yogurt, soaked Prunes and Figs, and Licorice tea.

Helpful foods: Brewers yeast, cabbage, cantaloupe, egg yolk, beef heart, brains, kidney, liver, rice bran, milk, nuts, peas, and soybeans.

Juices: Celery, grapefruit, and spinach juice.

LUMBAGO
(refer to Back Pain - page 103)

LUPUS

SPECIFICS: An inflammatory auto immune mechanism disease that affects many organs. Discoid lupus is a skin disease and systemic lupus affects the joints and organs of the body. Both types have remissions and flare up cycles.

(Beneficial Remedies, Treatments, and Nutrients)

Single herbs: Echinacea, Goldenseal, Pau d'Arco, Red Clover, Turkish Rhubarb, and Yucca.

Vitamins: C.

Minerals: Calcium, Magnesium, and Zinc.

Also: Canaid strengthens the immune system. Acidophilus, L-Cysteine, L-Cystine, L-Methionine, Proteolytic enzymes, and Unsaturated fatty acids.

Helpful foods: Broccoli, yellow corn, sweet potatoes, turnip greens, citrus fruits, cheese, butter, milk, shell fish, herring, and oysters.

LYME DISEASE

SPECIFICS: Lyme disease is caused by a tick that is carried by mice, lizards, and the white tailed deer. Tick bites often go undetected and the first sign of lyme disease is a rash a few days after the tick bite. Symptoms include backache, headache, stiff neck, nausea, and vomiting. If left untreated, lyme disease can lead to damage to the central nervous system and cardiovascular system.

(Beneficial Remedies, Treatments, and Nutrients)

Single herbs: Echinacea, Goldenseal, Milk thistle, Pau d'Arco, Red Clover, and Suma.

Vitamins: Multi-vitamin plus A, C, and E.

Minerals: Zinc.

Also: Chlorophyll and Germanium.

Helpful foods: Aloe Vera, broccoli, carrots, citrus fruits, garlic, vegetable oils, and fish liver oils.

MACULAR DEGENERATION

SPECIFICS: Macular degeneration is one of the leading causes of decreased visual acuity. This condition is characterized by the degeneration of the macula or the central area of the retina. Factors that contribute to the development of this disease include cigarette smoking, poor nutrition, hypertension, and atherosclerosis. Consumption of saturated fats, white sugar, and refined carbohydrates should be avoided.

(Beneficial Remedies, Treatments, and Nutrients)

Single herbs: Gingko Biloba, Bilberry, and Hawthorn.

Vitamins: A, Beta-carotene, C, and E.

Minerals: Selenium and Zinc.

Also: Bioflavonoids, Omega-3, and Omega-6.

Helpful foods: Broccoli, carrots, citrus fruits, garlic, strawberries, vegetable oils, and fish liver oils.

MALABSORPTION SYNDROME

SPECIFICS: This disorder is due to an incorrect diet over a long period of time. This condition will cause anemia and osteoporosis if not addressed in time. The problem is always due to malnutrition. Treatment is a diet high in all nutrients, vitamins, and minerals.

(Beneficial Remedies, Treatments, and Nutrients)

Single herbs: Kelp and Horsetail.

Vitamins: B12, B complex, and C.

Minerals: Multi-mineral complex plus Zinc.

Also: Acidophilus, Essential fatty acids, Liver, and Protein.

Helpful foods: All fruits(citrus and other), green leafy vegetables, turnip greens, nuts, unpolished rice, herring, oysters, and red meats.

Juices: Blackberry, grape, and parsley juice.

MANIC DEPRESSION

SPECIFICS: A mental disorder in which a disturbance of mood is the major symptom. Mood swings may be accompanied by extreme negative delusions or by grandiose ideas. The main causes of this ailment are drugs, inherited tendency, and malnutrition.

(Beneficial Remedies, Treatments, and Nutrients)

Vitamins: B complex, B12, and Folic Acid.

Minerals: Lithium.

Also: Omega-6 oils, L-phenylalanine, and L-tryptophan.

Helpful foods: Liver, red meat, eggs, asparagus, citrus fruits, turnip greens, sprouted seeds, cheese and other dairy products, sunflower seeds, wheat germ, and whole grains.

MARBLE BONE DISEASE

SPECIFICS: Marble bone disease is a gradual loss in the total mass of bone, leaving the remaining bone fragile or brittle. The major cause of this disease is a calcium-phosphorus imbalance or an inability to absorb sufficient amounts of calcium through the intestine. The best prevention and treatment is a diet that is adequate in vitamin C and D, protein, calcium, magnesium, and phosphorus.

(Beneficial Remedies, Treatments, and Nutrients)

Single herbs: Feverfew, Horsetail, and Oatstraw,

Vitamins: B12, C, D, and E.

Minerals: Calcium, Copper, Fluoride, Magnesium, and Phosphorus.

Also: L-Lysine, L-Arginine, Protein, Multidigestive enzymes with Betaine hydrochloride, and Proteolytic enzymes.

Helpful foods: All dairy products, red meats, chicken, sardines, tuna, herring, oysters, all fruit, soybeans, nuts, broccoli, corn, rice, and whole wheat.

MASTITIS *(Breast infection)*

SPECIFICS: Mastitis is the result of a plugged duct. If the mother should stop nursing the baby, the duct will remain full and could worsen the problem by allowing the duct to overfill. A few of the milder antibiotics can be taken while nursing. The following nutrients should be taken by the nursing mother.

(Beneficial Remedies, Treatments, and Nutrients)

Vitamins: A good multi-vitamin, plus B complex, C, and D.

Minerals: Calcium, Manganese, and Iron.

Also: Acidophlus and Protein.

Helpful foods: Tuna, red meat, beets, broccoli, peas, turnip greens, sprouted seeds, cheese and other dairy products, sunflower seeds, and whole rye.

MEASLES

SPECIFICS: The two main varieties of measles are German measles and common measles.

German measles is a contagious, but mild virus, however if contracted during the first four months of pregnancy it can cause serious birth defects.

Common measles may have many serious complications, such as bronchitis, croup, middle ear infection, or pneumonia.

(Beneficial Remedies, Treatments, and Nutrients)

HERBAL COMBINATION: (Fenu-Thyme) (ANT-PLG Syrup).

PHYSIOLOGIC ACTION: Helps the body to resist infectious diseases and reduce fever. Acts as a support to the immune system during such illnesses as chicken pox, mumps, and measles.

Single herbs: Garlic, Catnip tea, Turkey Rhubarb, and Pau d'Arco.

Vitamins: A, C, and E.

Minerals: Calcium, Magnesium, and Zinc.

Also: Canaid herbal drink helps to strengthen the immune system. Raw thymus and Proteolytic enzymes.

Helpful foods: Bananas, citrus fruits, melons, herring, fish liver oils, carrots, broccoli, green leafy vegetables, sweet potatoes, and turnip greens.

MELANOMA

SPECIFICS: The most dangerous form of skin cancer. Melanoma is life threatening, but can be cured if discovered and treated early. In this type of skin cancer, a tumor is produced from the pigment producing cells of the deeper layers of the skin. Most often it begins as a lesion that looks like a mole. The most common cause of melanoma is overexposure to the suns ultraviolet rays.

(Beneficial Remedies, Treatments, and Nutrients)

Single herbs: Kelp and Pau d'Arco.

Vitamins: A, B complex, B12, Niacin, Folic Acid, C, and E.

Minerals: A strong Multi-mineral plus Potassium, Calcium, and Magnesium.

Also: Coenzyme Q10, L-Cysteine, L-Methionine, L-Taurine, Essential fatty acids, Germanium, Primadophilus, Proteolytic enzymes, and Raw glandular complex with extra Raw thymus.

Helpful foods: Aloe Vera, apples, bananas, broccoli, bran, carrots, citrus fruits, green leafy vegetables, soybeans, sweet potatoes, turnip greens, vegetable oils, lean red meat, and fish liver oils.

MEMORY AID

SPECIFICS: Most memory lapses are caused by a deficiency of vitamins and minerals. Other causes may be due to cerebral dysfunction, nervous disturbances, and strokes.

(Beneficial Remedies, Treatments, and Nutrients)

HERBAL COMBINATIONS: (SEN) or (Remem).

PHYSIOLOGIC ACTION: This formula contains remarkable rejuvenating properties that nourish the brain cells and tissues and improves their ability to perform mental functions.

Single herbs: Cayenne, Ginkgo, Gotu Kola, Korean Ginseng, and Lobelia.

Vitamins: Multi-vitamin complex plus Choline.

Minerals: A good multi-mineral complex.

Also: Lecithin.

Helpful foods: Brewers yeast, egg yolk, green leafy vegetables, liver, and wheat germ.

MENIERE'S SYNDROME

SPECIFICS: A disease of the inner ear characterized by loss of hearing, ringing in the ears, nausea, vomiting, and dizziness. Meniere's syndrome is often caused by impaired blood flow to the brain from clogged arteries and poor circulation.

(Beneficial Remedies, Treatments, and Nutrients)

HERBAL COMBINATIONS: (H Formula) (Ginkgold).

PHYSIOLOGIC ACTION: Contains herbs which strengthen the heart and builds the vascular system. When taken with Cayenne, it improves circulation and pulse rate, giving a warming sensation to the entire body.

Single herbs: Cayenne, Black Cohosh, Bayberry, Butchers Broom, Ginkgo, and Yarrow

Vitamins: A, B complex, B3, B6, C, and E.

Minerals: Calcium, Magnesium, Manganese, and Potassium.

Also: Bio-Strath, Coenzyme Q10, and Lecithin.

Helpful foods: All vegetables and vegetable oils, apples, bananas, citrus fruits, beets, broccoli, carrots, oat bran, soya beans, and whole wheat.

MENINGITIS

SPECIFICS: This disease occurs when the three layers of membranes lying between the skull and the brain, called the "meninges", become infected. Medical attention should be sought promptly, if untreated complications such as brain damage and paralysis can occur.
Symptoms include drowsiness, chills, high fever, headache, nausea, and a stiff neck. A well-balanced diet high in vitamins, minerals, and protein will help the body ward off infection and repair damaged tissue.

(Beneficial Remedies, Treatments, and Nutrients)

Single herbs: Catnip and Garlic.

Vitamins: Multi-vitamin plus A, C, and D.

Minerals: A high potency mineral complex, Calcium, and Zinc.

Also: Germanium, Protein, and Raw thymus.

Helpful foods: Aloe Vera juice, butter, cheese and other dairy products, citrus fruit, tuna, beef, sardines, herring, oysters, and sweet potatoes.

MENOPAUSE

SPECIFICS: Menopause is the point at which women stop ovulating, the end of their reproductive years. It usually lasts from three to five years and is experienced by most women around the age of fifty. Symptoms include difficult breathing, dizziness, headache, heart palpitations, hot flashes, and depression.

(Beneficial Remedies, Treatments, and Nutrients)

HERBAL COMBINATIONS: (Change-O-Life) or (MP).

PHYSIOLOGIC ACTION: For both male and female health to the pancreas, pituitary, and other glandular areas. Maintains a healthy hormone balance in the body, especially during puberty and menopause.

Single herbs: Black Cohosh, Blessed Thistle, Damiana, Licorice Root, Quan Yin, Sarsaparilla, and Siberian Ginseng,

HOMEOPATHIC COMBINATION: Menopause Formula.

Vitamins: A, B complex, B3, C, D, and E.

Minerals: Calcium, Magnesium, Potassium, and Selenium.

Also: Enzymes with hydrochloric acid, Germanium, L-Arginine, L-Lysine, and Melbrosia.

Helpful foods: All vegetables and vegetable oils, fish and fish liver oils, cheese, butter, apples, bananas, citrus fruits, and mushrooms.

MENSTRUATION

SPECIFICS: Menstruation is the cyclical process that continuously
prepares the uterus for pregnancy, starting at puberty and continuing through menopause.

(Beneficial Remedies, Treatments, and Nutrients)

HERBAL COMBINATIONS: (FC) or (FEM-MEND).

PHYSIOLOGIC ACTION: Helps regulate the menstrual cycle, relieve cramps, bloating and vaginitis, ease inflammation of the
vagina and uterus, and strengthen and regulate the kidneys, bladder and uterus areas. Beneficial for all female and uterine complaints.

WARNING: Do not use this combination while taking estrogen or oral contraceptives!

Single herbs: Red Raspberry and Uva Ursi.

HOMEOPATHIC COMBINATION: PMS Formula.

Vitamins: B complex, B6, C, E.

Minerals: A complete multi-mineral.

Helpful foods: Dulse, pineapples, citrus fruits, broccoli, soybeans, spinach, sweet potatoes, turnip greens, vegetable oils, nuts, unpolished rice, and whole wheat.

MENSTRUAL CRAMPS
(refer to Premenstrual Syndrome - PMS - page 134)

MERCURY POISONING

SPECIFICS: Mercury is found in the soil, water, our food supply and is even more toxic than lead. It is accumulated and retained in the brain and central nervous system. Large amounts of mercury can cause depression, dizziness, fatigue, memory loss and weakness.

(Beneficial Remedies, Treatments, and Nutrients)

Single herbs: Alfalfa, Kelp, and Garlic.

PHYSIOLOGIC ACTION: Garlic acts as a detoxifier and alfalfa and kelp help the body to remove the toxins.

Vitamins: A, B complex, C, and E.

Minerals: Selenium.

Also: L-Cysteine, L- Cystine, L- Glutathione, L- Methionine, and Hydrochloric acid.

Helpful foods: Apples, garlic, onions, fruit and vegetable juices, oat bran, and whole grains.

MIGRAINE HEADACHES

SPECIFICS: A migraine headache begins with a throbbing pain that usually begins at the back of the head and spreads to the entire side of the head or is centered above or behind one eye. Most migraines are caused by allergies, constipation, stress, or liver malfunction. Note - Avoid the following: salt, dairy products, red meat, and fried foods.

(Beneficial Remedies, Treatments, and Nutrients)

Single herbs: Chamomile, Feverfew, Ginkgo Biloba, and Yucca.

PHYSIOLOGIC ACTION: Chamomile will prevent migraine headaches. Ginkgo Biloba enhances cerebral circulation. Feverfew reduces fever. Feverfew has been historically used for chills and pain that accompany fever. Because of its anecdotal claims for migraine sufferers, it is presently being researched at the London Migraine Clinic.

HOMEOPATHIC COMBINATION: Migraine Headache Formula.

Vitamins: B complex, B3, B5, B12, Paba, and Niacin, C, and F.

Minerals: Calcium, Magnesium, and Potassium.

Also: Unsaturated fatty acids.

Helpful foods: Almonds, apples, avocados, bananas, all vegetables and vegetable oils, citrus fruits, whole grains, and unpolished rice.

MITRAL VALVE PROLAPSE

SPECIFICS: A mitral valve prolapse is a common condition that is usually detected if a heart murmer and/or click is heard, and is generally considered a benign heart valve abnormality.

(Beneficial Remedies, Treatments, and Nutrients)

Vitamins: Multi-vitamin.

Minerals: Multi-mineral plus extra Magnesium.

Also: Coenzyme Q10.

MONONUCLEOSIS

SPECIFICS: An infectious disease believed to be caused by a virus. It affects the respiratory system, liver, the lymph tissues, and glands. The disease can be transmitted through communal drinking utensils, kissing , and blood transfusions. A well-balanced diet, adequate in protein, is essential for the prevention of mononucleosis.

(Beneficial Remedies, Treatments, and Nutrients)

Single herbs: Dandelion, Echinacea, Goldenseal, Pau d'Arco, and Sheep Sorrel.

Vitamins: A, B complex, B1, B2, B5, B6, C, Biotin, and Choline.

Minerals: Potassium.

Also: Canaid herbal drink, a nondairy form of Acidophilus, Germanium, Raw thymus, Raw glandular complex, and Protein.

Helpful foods: Aloe Vera, bananas, melons, citrus fruits, nuts, oat bran, green leafy vegetables, sweet potatoes, turnip greens, carrots, and fish liver oils.

MORNING SICKNESS

SPECIFICS: About half of all pregnant women experience nausea and vomiting from the 5th week to the 12th week of pregnancy. Morning sickness may be due to either a dairy product intolerance or a nutrient deficiency.

(Beneficial Remedies, Treatments, and Nutrients)

Single herbs: Red Raspberry and Peppermint.

PHYSIOLOGIC ACTION: Red Raspberry or Peppermint Tea often overcomes nausea. Alfalfa, Chamomile, Catnip, and Ginger tea may also be helpful. Sometimes small, frequent meals instead of a larger one is beneficial.

Vitamins: A multi-vitamin plus B6, C, and K.

Also: Eliminate alcohol from your diet. Avoid cigarette smoke, yours and other people's. Do not use white sugar, refined carbohydrates, coffee and other stimulants.

Helpful foods: Broccoli, kale, lettuce, spinach, turnip greens, and strawberries.

MOTION SICKNESS

SPECIFICS: Motion induced nausea can indicate the presence of many diseases including inner ear infection, low blood sugar, food poisoning, and nutrient deficiency. The most common cause is a deficiency of the vitamin "B6" and the mineral "magnesium". Ginkgo is excellent for chronic dizziness and light headedness.
Natural remedies have been used with great success in cases of motion sickness. Do not eat junk foods, heavily processed meals, or alcohol before or during the trip.

(Beneficial Remedies, Treatments, and Nutrients)

HERBAL COMBINATION: (Motion Mate).

PHYSIOLOGIC ACTION: In a recent university study, ginger root caps proved more effective than either a drug or placebo at controlling motion induced nausea. Also queasy travelers have found taking B complex at night and just before the trip is most effective.

Single herbs: Ginger Root Caps and Ginkgo.

Vitamins: B complex, plus B6.

Minerals: Magnesium.

Also: Charcoal tablets.

Helpful foods: Fruits, lean beef, nuts, unpolished rice, whole grains, and yellow corn.

MOUTH AND TONGUE DISORDERS
(Canker, Thrush, Pyorrhea)

SPECIFICS: Nearly all mouth and tongue disorders such as sore mouth, tongue, and gums are attributed to a deficiency of the B vitamins. The gums become puffy, tender, and the oral membranes become susceptible to canker sores with the deficiency of vitamin C and niacin.

(Beneficial Remedies, Treatments, and Nutrients)

Single herbs: Aloe Vera, Golden Seal, Myrrh, Red Raspberry, and White Oak Bark.

Vitamins: A, B complex, B2, B3, B12, C, and E.

Minerals: Iron, Magnesium, Phosphorus, and Zinc.

Also: Chlorophyll, Lysine, and Primadophilus.

Helpful foods: All fruits, carrots, corn, broccoli, herring, oysters, red meat, soybeans, and spinach.

MULTIPLE SCLEROSIS

SPECIFICS: MS is a degenerative and progressive disorder of the central nervous system that destroys the myelin sheaths which cover the nerves, causing an inflammatory response. A strong immune system helps avoid infection and a diet rich in vitamin and mineral supplements is beneficial for the MS patient.

Note: Limit the consumption of saturated fats, sugar, and processed foods.

(Beneficial Remedies, Treatments, and Nutrients)

Single herbs: Evening Primrose Oil, Kelp, Oat Extract, Skullcap, and St. John's Wort.

Vitamins: B complex, B1, B2, B3, B5, B6, B12, C, E, F, and Inositol.

Minerals: Calcium, Copper, Iron, Magnesium, Manganese, Selenium, and Zinc.

Also: Acidophilus, Bonemeal, Coenzyme Q10, Germanium, Digestive enzymes, Proteolytic enzymes, Lecithin, L-Leucine, L-Isoleucine, L-Valine, and Protein.

Helpful foods: Apples, apricots, cherries, grapes, citrus fruits, cheese, beets, broccoli, green leafy vegetables, soy beans, spinach, red meat, mushrooms, and garlic.

MUMPS

SPECIFICS: A contagious viral infection that causes swelling of one or both parotid glands at the jaw angles below the ears. Mumps usually infect children between the ages of three and twelve, however they can occur after puberty and cause serious complications such as sterility in the ovaries and testes.

(Beneficial Remedies, Treatments, and Nutrients)

HERBAL COMBINATION: (ANT-PLG).

PHYSIOLOGIC ACTION: An effective formula that helps cleanse toxins and reduce infection. This combination is a natural aid in fighting contagious diseases.

Single herbs: Bayberry Root Bark, Echinacea, Ginger Root, Lobelia, and Mullein.

Vitamins: A, B complex, C, and E.

Minerals: A complete multi complex.

Also: Germanium and Acidophilus.

Helpful foods: Bananas, citrus fruits, melons, herring, fish liver oils, carrots, broccoli, green leafy vegetables, sweet potatoes, and turnip greens.

MUSCLE CRAMPS

SPECIFICS: An involuntary spasm or contraction of the muscle. Most cramps occur at night after a day of unusual exertion, when the limbs are cool. Muscle cramps are caused by impaired blood circulation or a calcium and magnesium imbalance.

(Beneficial Remedies, Treatments, and Nutrients)

HERBAL COMBINATION: (Ca-T).

PHYSIOLOGIC ACTION: Effectively calms nerves and aids sleep in addition to rebuilding the nerve sheath, vein, and artery walls.

Single herbs: Comfrey Herb, Dong Quai, Elderberry, Ginkgo Biloba, Horsetail Grass, Oat Straw, Saffron, and Skullcap.

Vitamins: A, B complex, B1, B3, B5, C, D, and E.

Minerals: Calcium, Magnesium, and Zinc.

Also: #12 tissue salts, Coenzyme Q10, and Lecithin.

Helpful foods: Red meat, butter, cheese, citrus fruits, soybeans, rice, sunflower seeds, nuts, whole grains, and sweet potatoes.

MUSCLE INJURIES
(refer to Athletic Injuries - page 16)

MUSCLE WEAKNESS

SPECIFICS: Almost every nutrient is involved in muscle contraction, relaxation, and repair. A deficiency interferes with the metabolism of amino acids and increases the need for oxygen in the blood. This in turn, causes a gradual, progressive weakness throughout the muscles of the body.

(Beneficial Remedies, Treatments, and Nutrients)

Single herbs: Gota Kola and Ginseng.

Vitamins: A complete multi-vitamin plus additional E.

Minerals: Manganese, Potassium, and Zinc.

Also: Protein and Unsaturated fatty acids.

Helpful foods: All vegetables and vegetable oils, bananas, herring, oysters, and whole wheat.

MUSCULAR DYSTROPHY

SPECIFICS: In muscular dystrophy the essential fatty acids that form the structural part of the muscle are destroyed and the nutrients necessary for muscle function are reduced. The disease is considered to be largely hereditary, except for one type that occurs in adults between the ages of forty to fifty. The victims diet should be adequate in all essential nutrients including proteins and vegetable oils.

(Beneficial Remedies, Treatments, and Nutrients)

Single herbs: Saw Palmetto.

Vitamins: A, B complex, B3, B5, B6, B12, C, E, and Choline.

Minerals: Potassium.

Also: Protein and Unsaturated fatty acids.

Helpful foods: All fruits, all vegetables and vegetable oils, whole grains and seeds, red meat, sardines, herring, oysters, and fish liver oils.

MYALGIA
(refer to Muscle Cramps - page 115)

MYASTHENIA GRAVIS

SPECIFICS: Myasthenia usually effects muscles in the face and neck. This disease is caused by underproduction of acetylcholine, a substance that transmits nerve impulses to the muscles. Many nutrients are required for the production of acetylcholine, and in many cases recovery from the ailment has occurred with the use of a proper diet.

(Beneficial Remedies, Treatments, and Nutrients)

Single herbs: Dong Quai and Korean Ginseng.

Vitamins: B complex, B1, B2, B6, B12, Choline, Folic acid, Inositol, Pantothenic acid, C, and E.

Minerals: Magnesium, Manganese, and Potassium.

Also: Lecithin and Protein.

Helpful foods: Apples, bananas, grapes, citrus fruits, beets, broccoli, yellow corn, soybeans, and nuts.

MYCOSES

SPECIFICS: Diseases of the skin or other organs caused by the multiplication and spread of fungi. Victims of mycoses should eat a well-balanced diet, supplemented by megadoses of vitamins A, B, and C.

(Beneficial Remedies, Treatments, and Nutrients)

Single herbs: Black Walnut, Garlic, and Pau d'Arco.

Vitamins: A, B, C, and E.

Also: Primadophilus and Caprinex.

Helpful foods: Beef, chicken, tuna, carrots, black walnut, raw fruits, spinach, turnip greens, and sweet potatoes.

<u>Note:</u> Avoid dairy products and processed foods.

MYOCARDIAL INFARCTION

SPECIFICS: When the heart is temporarily deprived of oxygen due to the thickening, hardening, and narrowing of the coronary arteries. A coronary may be triggered by complete or partial blockage of the coronary arteries. Recent animal studies suggest that vitamin C deficiency could, be involved in the causation of myocardial infarction. E.F.A.s (essential fatty acids) play a fundamental role in keeping cell membranes, fluid and flexible.

(Beneficial Remedies, Treatments, and Nutrients)

HERBAL COMBINATION: (Garlicin HC).

PHYSIOLOGIC ACTION: A combination of herbs which supports the cardiovascular system. Helps to strengthen the heart, while building and cleansing the arteries and veins.

Single herbs: Cayenne, Comfrey, Evening Primrose Oil, Fish Oil, Garlic, Golden Seal, and Rose Hips.

Vitamins: B complex, C, E, Niacin, Inositol, and Choline.

Minerals: Calcium and Magnesium

Also: Coenzyme Q10, L-Carnitine, L-Cysteine, L-Methionine, Multidigestive enzymes, DMG, Fish oils, and cold pressed vegetable oils.

Helpful foods: Apples, lean beef, broccoli, fruits(citrus and other),sprouted seeds, sunflower seeds, sweet potatoes, sardines, tuna, turnip greens, and yellow corn.

NAIL PROBLEMS

SPECIFICS: Nail changes or abnormalities are often the result of nutritional deficiencies. A well-balanced diet supplying all essential nutrients is recommended.

Vitamin A deficiency causes dryness and brittleness.

Vitamin B deficiency causes fragility.

Vitamin C deficiency causes hangnails.

Iron deficiency causes thinning and flattening.

Zinc deficiency causes white spots.

(Beneficial Remedies, Treatments, and Nutrients)

Single herbs: Horsetail.

Vitamins: A, B complex, and C.

Minerals: Calcium, Magnesium, Iron, and Zinc.

Also: L-Cysteine, L-Methionine, Protein, and Silicon.

Helpful foods: All dairy products, red meat, chicken, tuna, salmon, sardines, all vegetables, and vegetable oils.

Juices: Beet greens, celery, kale, and parsley juice.

NAUSEA AND VOMITING

SPECIFICS: Both illnesses can indicate the presence of one of many diseases, and both are produced by a deficiency of magnesium and/or vitamin B6.

(Beneficial Remedies, Treatments, and Nutrients)

HERBAL COMBINATION: (Herbal Influence).

PHYSIOLOGIC ACTION: Herbal Influence (formerly known as Herbal Composition) was created by the early American herbalist, Samuel Thomson. It contains herbs which help with fever and nauseousness.

Single herbs: Cayenne, Red Clover, Raspberry Tea, Chaparral, Rose Hips, Garlic, Honey, and Golden Seal.

Vitamins: A, B6, C, and P.

Minerals: Magnesium.

Helpful foods: Apples, apricots, avocados, citrus fruits, broccoli, carrots, peas, sweet potatoes, turnip greens, yellow corn, red meats, rice, and buck wheat.

Juices: Carrot and blackberry juice.

NEPHRITIS
(refer to Kidney and Bladder - page 96)

(refer to Kidney and Bladder - page 96)

NERVOUS DISORDERS

SPECIFICS: Nervous disorders are generally a direct result of stress. The body can handle some stress but long term stress causes the body to break down. Long term stress occurs when the situation that causes anxiety is not relieved. Find the cause and handle it constructively. People experiencing stress should maintain a well-balanced diet and replace the nutrients depleted during stress.

(Beneficial Remedies, Treatments, and Nutrients)

HERBAL COMBINATIONS: (Calm-aid) or (Ex stress comb).

PHYSIOLOGIC ACTION: A proven formula that is soothing, strengthening, and healing to the whole nervous system to relieve nervous tension and rebuild the nerve sheaths. Excellent aid for insomnia, chronic nervousness, and stress-related conditions.

Single herbs: Evening Primrose Oil, Hops, Mistletoe, Skullcap, Valerian, and Yucca.

Vitamins: B complex, B1, B2, B3, B5, B6, and C.

Minerals: Calcium, Iodine, Iron, Magnesium, Phosphorus, Potassium, Silicon, and Sodium.

Helpful foods: Dulse, flax seed, sea salt, fruit(citrus and other), bacon, beef, chicken, all dairy products, all vegetables, and whole rye.

Juices: Radish and prune juice.

NETTLE RASH

SPECIFICS: If the sap of nettles touches the skin, it can cause persistent itching, rash, swelling, and blistering in sensitive people. The following nutrients will help alleviate the symptoms.

(Beneficial Remedies, Treatments, and Nutrients)

Single herbs: Echinacea, Goldenseal, and Lobelia.

Vitamins: A, C, and E.

Minerals: Zinc.

Helpful foods: Broccoli, carrots, citrus fruits, melon, fish liver oils, and vegetable oils.

NEURITIS

SPECIFICS: Neuritis is the inflammation or deterioration of a nerve or a group of nerves. It is caused by an injury to a nerve, diabetes, infection, or the deficiency of the vitamin B complex. The best treatment for neuritis is to make sure the patient gets optimum nutrition.

(Beneficial Remedies, Treatments, and Nutrients)

Single herbs: Black Cohosh, Lobelia, Lady Slipper, Skullcap, and Valerian Root.

Vitamins: B1, B2, B6, B12, Niacin, and Pantothenic acid.

Minerals: Mineral complex, plus Calcium and Magnesium.

Also: Lecithin, Protein, and Proteolytic enzymes.

Helpful foods: Brewers yeast, cheese, all fruit, nuts, oat bran, and unpolished rice.

Juices: Cucumber, Endive, and Pineapple juice.

NIGHT BLINDNESS

SPECIFICS: The inability to see well in dim light. The condition may be an inherited functional defect of the retina but the most common cause is a deficiency of vitamin A. Night blindness can usually be prevented by supplementing the diet with vitamins and the nutrients listed.

(Beneficial Remedies, Treatments, and Nutrients)

HERBAL COMBINATION: (Herbal Eye bright Formula).

PHYSIOLOGIC ACTION: Extremely valuable in strengthening and healing the eyes. Aids the body in healing lesions and eye injuries.

WARNING: If symptoms persist, discontinue use.

Also: The herb eye bright may be used as a wash for superficial inflammations of the eye.

Single herbs: Bilberry, and Eyebright.

Vitamins: A Multi-vitamin complex, plus A, B1, B2, B3, B5, B6, C D, and E.

Minerals: Calcium, Copper, Manganese, Magnesium, Potassium, Selenium, and Zinc.

Also: Gyncydo, and Protein.

Helpful foods: Apples, citrus fruits, beets, rice bran, carrots, green leafy vegetables, herring, oysters, red meat, chicken, nuts, and soybeans.

NOCTURIA

SPECIFICS: The disturbance of a person's sleep by the need to pass urine. Common causes are infection, cystitis (inflammation of the bladder), and enlargement of the prostate gland (obstructs the normal outflow of urine and causes the bladder to empty incompletely). Rarer causes of nocturia include diabetes insipidus, diabetes mellitus, and chronic kidney failure.

(Beneficial Remedies, Treatments, and Nutrients)

HERBAL COMBINATION: (KB).

PHYSIOLOGIC ACTION: Extremely valuable in healing and strengthening the kidneys, bladder, and genito-urinary area. Useful to stop bed-wetting, but is a diuretic when congestion of the kidneys is indicated. Helps remove bladder, uterine, and urethral toxins.

WARNING: Intended for occasional use only. May cause green-yellow discoloration of urine.

Single herbs: Alfalfa, Barberry root, Catnip, Dandelion, Fennel, Ginger root, Goldenrod, Horsetail, Uva Ursi, and Wild Yam.

Vitamins: A, B complex, C, D, E, and Choline.

Minerals: Calcium, Magnesium, and Potassium.

Also: Digestive enzymes, Lecithin, L-Arginine, L-Methionine, Propolis, Uratonic, Watermelon, 3-way herb teas, and other Diuretic tablets.

Helpful foods: All vegetables, apples, bananas, broccoli, carrots, cheese and other dairy products, tuna, and fish liver oils, red meat, and sprouted seeds.

Juices: Asparagus, black currant, cranberry, celery, juniper berry, parsley, and pomegranate juice.

NUTRITIONAL DISORDERS

SPECIFICS: Nutritional disorders are usually caused by a deficiency or excess of one or more of the elements of nutrition. Inadequate intake of protein and calories may occur in individuals that have an intense fear of becoming obese. Recent studies show that some nutritional disorders may be caused by a severe zinc deficiency. When trying to stimulate the appetite, consider the aroma and appearance of foods, as well as the nutritional value.

(Beneficial Remedies, Treatments, and Nutrients)

Single herbs: Catnip, Fennel, Ginger, Ginseng, Gotu Kola, Kelp, Papaya, Peppermint, and Saw Palmetto.

Vitamins: Multi-vitamins plus A, B12, B complex, D, and E.

Minerals: Multi-minerals plus Potassium, Selenium, and Zinc.

Also: Acidophilus, Bio-Strath, Brewer's yeast, Liver, Protein, and Proteolytic enzymes.

Helpful foods: Butter, bran, beef, bananas, herring, sunflower seeds, soybeans, spinach, tuna, and nuts.

OBESITY

SPECIFICS: A person who has twenty percent excess body fat over the norm for their age, build, and height is considered obese. Losing weight is a matter of consciously regulating the types and amount of food eaten and increasing daily activity. Some hormonal disorders are accompanied by obesity, but the overwhelming majority of obese people do not suffer from such disorders.

(Beneficial Remedies, Treatments, and Nutrients)

HERBAL COMBINATIONS: (SKC) or (Herbal Slim).

PHYSIOLOGIC ACTION: This effective formula cleanses the bowels and eliminates excess water. Helps control appetite, dissolves excess fat, reduces tension, stress, and anxiety associated with dieting.

Single herbs: Chickweed, Hawthorn Berries, Kelp, Licorice Root, Papaya Leaves, Saffron, and Yucca.

Vitamins: B2, B5, B6, B12, B complex, C, E, Choline, Folic Acid, Inositol, and Pantothenic acid.

Minerals: Calcium, Magnesium, and Phosphorus.

Also: Yu-ccan herbal drink, Lecithin, Protein, and Unsaturated fatty acids.

Helpful foods: Shell fish, white meat of chicken, tuna, citrus fruits, green leafy vegetables, and sprouted seeds.

Juices: Beet greens, Celery, and Parsley juice.

OPTIC NEURITIS

SPECIFICS: Optic neuritis is the inflammation or deterioration of the optic nerve in the eye, causing gradual or sudden blurred vision. The eye may be painful and temporary blindness may occur in severe cases. The best treatment for optic neuritis is to make sure the patient gets rest and optimum nutrition.

(Beneficial Remedies, Treatments, and Nutrients)

Single herbs: Black Cohosh, Lobelia, Lady Slipper, Skullcap, and Valerian Root.

Vitamins: B1, B2, B6, B12, Niacin, and Pantothenic acid.

Minerals: Mineral complex plus Calcium and Magnesium.

Also: Lecithin, Protein, and Proteolytic enzymes.

Helpful foods: All dairy products, beef, yellow corn, fruit, nuts, oat bran, and unpolished rice.

OSTEOARTHRITIS

SPECIFICS: Osteoarthritis is a degenerative joint disease involving the deterioration of the cartilage at the ends of the bones, causing the cartilage to become rough resulting in friction. This form of arthritis usually affects the weight bearing joints, such as the hips and knees.

(Beneficial Remedies, Treatments, and Nutrients)

HERBAL COMBINATION: (Rheum-Aid) or (Yucca -AR).

PHYSIOLOGIC ACTION: Relieves symptoms associated with bursitis, calcification, gout, rheumatoid arthritis, rheumatism, and osteoarthritis. Helps the body reduce or eliminate swelling and inflammation in the joints and connective tissue. Also helps to relieve stiffness and pain.

Single herbs: Alfalfa, Black Cohosh, Burdock, Cayenne, Celery seed, Chaparral, Devil's Claw, Valerian root, and Yucca.

Vitamins: Niacin, B5, B6, B12, B complex, C, D, E, F, and P.

Minerals: A strong Multi-mineral complex plus Calcium and Magnesium.

Also: Cod liver oil, Green Magma, Aqua life, Seatone, Bromelain, Goats milk, and Mung beans.

Helpful foods: Almonds, apples, apricots, avocados, cherries, broccoli, soybeans, spinach, sprouted seeds, sweet potatoes, buckwheat, whole wheat, red meat, citrus fruit, and all dairy products.

Juices: Cherry, papaya, and pineapple juice.

OSTEOMALACIA

SPECIFICS: A disease of malnutrition caused by a deficiency of calcium, phosphorus, and vitamin D. This causes the bones to become soft, resulting in deformities. It is most likely to occur at times of body stress, when pregnant, or breast feeding.

(Beneficial Remedies, Treatments, and Nutrients)

Single herbs: Horsetail.

Vitamins: A, B12, C, and D.

Minerals: Calcium, Magnesium, and Phosphorus.

Also: Cod liver oil, Lecithin, Hydrochloric acid, Silica, and Digestive enzymes.

Helpful foods: Beef, butter, cheese, tuna, fish liver oils, green leafy vegetables, turnip greens, fruit(citrus and other), nuts, and sunflower seeds.

OSTEOPOROSIS *(Brittle bones)*

SPECIFICS: Osteoporosis is a gradual loss in the total mass of bone, leaving the remaining bone fragile or brittle. The major cause of osteoporosis is a calcium-phosphorus imbalance or an inability to absorb sufficient amounts of calcium through the intestine. The best prevention and treatment is a diet that is adequate in vitamin C and D, protein, calcium, magnesium, and phosphorus.

(Beneficial Remedies, Treatments, and Nutrients)

Single herbs: Feverfew, Horsetail, and Oatstraw,

Vitamins: B12, C, D, and E.

Minerals: Calcium, Copper, Fluoride, Magnesium, and Phosphorus.

Also: L-Lysine, L-Arginine, Protein, Multidigestive enzymes with Betaine hydrochloride, and Proteolytic enzymes.

Helpful foods: All dairy products, red meats, chicken, sardines, tuna, herring, oysters, all fruit, soybeans, nuts, broccoli, corn, rice, and whole wheat.

OTITIS EXTERNA

SPECIFICS: The most common type of ear infection, also known as swimmers ear. This ailment is caused by generalized infection causing inflammation of the outer ear canal. Symptoms of the infection are fever, severe pain, and discharge from the ear.

(Beneficial Remedies, Treatments, and Nutrients)

HERBAL COMBINATIONS: (ImmunAid) (B&B Extract) (EchinaGuard).

PHYSIOLOGIC ACTION: ImmunAid boosts immunity, thereby helping with ear infections. EchinaGuard is a liquid and Echinacea extract is excellent for small children with ear infections. B&B Extract can be placed in the ear or taken internally. It is also used to aid poor equilibrium, and nervous conditions.

Single herbs: Blue Cohosh, Echinacea, Garlic Oil, Garlic, Mullein Oil, Mullein, Skullcap, Sheep Sorrel, and St. John's Wort.

HOMEOPATHIC COMBINATION: Earache Formula.

Vitamins: A, B complex, and C.

Minerals: Calcium and Zinc.

Also: Canaid herbal drink, Propolis, Protein, and Primadophilus. When combating ear infections, it is imperative to exclude allergen foods from the diet. This is particularly true of all dairy products.

Helpful foods: Lean red meat, carrots, green vegetables, citrus fruits, fish liver oils, herring, oysters, sardines, nuts, sprouted seeds, and sunflower seeds.

PAIN (Headaches, Tension)

SPECIFICS: Pain is a localized sensation that can range from mild discomfort to an excruciating and unbearable experience. It is the result of stimulation of special sensory nerve endings usually following injury or caused by disease.

(Beneficial Remedies, Treatments, and Nutrients)

HERBAL COMBINATION: (A-P).

PHYSIOLOGIC ACTION: Helps relieve pain in any part of the body. A natural way to ease chronic pain, headaches, childbirth after-pains, aching teeth, nervous tension, spasms, and intestinal gas.

Single herbs: Pau d'Arco.

HOMEOPATHIC COMBINATION: Tension Headache Formula.

Minerals: Calcium.

Also: DLPA (amino acid), and Lobelia.

Helpful foods: All dairy products, beef, cod liver oil, tuna, beets, broccoli, carrot, celery, peanuts, sunflower seeds, soybeans, and sprouted seeds.

Juices: Carrot, celery, lettuce, and tomato juice.

PANCREATITIS

SPECIFICS: An inflammation of the pancreas, caused by an obstruction of the pancreatic duct from cancer scarring or stones. The pancreas secretes insulin and digestive enzymes, and for this reason pancreatitis often causes diabetes and digestive disorders.

(Beneficial Remedies, Treatments, and Nutrients)

HERBAL COMBINATION: (PC).

PHYSIOLOGIC ACTION: Helps eliminate mucus and sedimentation, arrest infection, and stimulate and restore the natural functions of the pancreas. Also used for blood-sugar problems and healing the spleen.

Single herbs: Dandelion, Golden Seal, Juniper Berries, and Uva Ursi.

Vitamins: A, B complex, C, E, Choline, and Inositol.

Minerals: Chromium, Potassium, and Zinc.

Also: Coenzyme Q10, Germanium, Lecithin, Proteolytic enzymes, and Raw pancreas concentrate.

Helpful foods: All vegetables, vegetable oils, bananas, citrus fruits, herring, oysters, shellfish, fish liver oils, soybeans, and spinach.

Juices: Beet root and radish juice.

PARASITES

SPECIFICS: Parasites live in the gastrointestinal tract. Early signs include diarrhea, loss of appetite, and rectal itching.

If not eliminated they will result in the loss of weight, colon disorders, and anemia. Causes include ingestion of eggs or larvae from partially cooked meat, improper disposal of human waste, and walking barefoot on contaminated soil.

(Beneficial Remedies, Treatments, and Nutrients)

HERBAL COMBINATIONS: (Para-X) (Para-VF).

PHYSIOLOGIC ACTION: Useful in destroying and eliminating parasites, such as worms. Also helps relieve many kinds of skin problems. The Para-VF is liquid and is useful for children and the elderly who cannot swallow capsules.

WARNING: Do not use during pregnancy!

Single herbs: Black Walnut, Garlic, Pumpkin Seeds, Sage, Sheep Sorrel, Swedish Bitters, and Wormwood.

Vitamins: Folic Acid.

Minerals: A multi-mineral complex.

CHILDREN: Chamomile tea or raisins soaked in Senna tea for older children may be helpful.

Helpful foods: Asparagus, brewers yeast, broccoli, lettuce, lima beans, liver, mushrooms, nuts, and spinach.

PARKINSONS DISEASE

SPECIFICS: A degenerative disease affecting the nervous system that causes muscle tremor, stiffness, and weakness. The cause of the disease is unknown, but malnutrition is believed to be a major underlying factor. A low protein diet of raw, organic foods is best for patients with Parkinson's Disease.

(Beneficial Remedies, Treatments, and Nutrients)

Single herbs: Ginseng, Damiana, and Cayenne

Vitamins: B complex, plus B2, B6, C, and E.

Minerals: Calcium Lactate, and Magnesium.

Also: Brewer's yeast, Lecithin, Multidigestive enzymes, L-Glutamic acid, and L-Tyrosine.

Helpful foods: Apples, apricots, cherries, grapes, citrus fruits, oat bran, broccoli, carrots, yellow corn, vegetable oils, and unpolished rice

PELLAGRA

SPECIFICS: A vitamin deficiency disease, caused by the long term shortage of B vitamins. A diet with niacin, thiamine, riboflavin, folic acid, and vitamin B12 will cure the disease.

(Beneficial Remedies, Treatments, and Nutrients)

Vitamins: B complex, plus extra B1, B2, B3, B12, and Folic acid.

Minerals: Calcium and Zinc.

Also: Protein and Tryptophan.

Helpful foods: Avocados, bananas, broccoli, figs, legumes, nuts, potatoes, tomatoes, and prunes.

Juices: Blackberry, grape, and parsley juice.

PEPTIC ULCERS

SPECIFICS: Peptic ulcers occur along the gastrointestinal tract and result when, during stress, the stomach is unable to secrete sufficient mucus, to protect against the strong acid essential for digestion. Symptoms of an ulcer are choking sensations, nausea, lower back pain, and stomach pain. Most ulcers are aggravated by the level of anxiety of the individual before eating.

(Beneficial Remedies, Treatments, and Nutrients)

HERBAL COMBINATION: (Myrrh – Gold Seal Plus).

Single herbs: Cayenne (stomach ulcers only), Golden Seal, Myrrh, Pau d'Arco, Red Raspberry, Slippery Elm Bark, Valerian, and White Oak Bark.

Vitamins: A, B complex, B2, B5, B6, B12, C, D, E, P, Choline, and Folic acid.

Minerals: Calcium, Manganese, and Zinc,

Also: Acidophilus, Adrenal glandular extract, Bioflavonoids, Bromelain, Chlorophyll, Raw Cabbage, Glutamine, Goat's milk, Brewer's yeast, and Halibut oil.

Refer to "Digestive Disorders" in this manual.

Helpful foods: Avocados, bananas, green leafy vegetables, red meat, bacon, chicken, cheese, fish liver oils, vegetable oils, oat bran, and whole grains.

Juices: Aloe Vera, celery, grapefruit, potato, and spinach juice.

PERIODONTITIS

SPECIFICS: Periodontitis(a gum disease) accounts for the loss of more teeth than cavities.

Periodontitis is an inflammation of the bones and gums that surround and support the teeth. This disease is caused by improper cleaning of teeth and gums, poorly fitting dentures, loose fillings, or an inadequate diet.

(Beneficial Remedies, Treatments, and Nutrients)

Single herbs: Chamomile, Echinacea, Lobelia, Myrrh Gum, and White Oak Bark.

Vitamins: A, B complex, C, D, P, Niacin, and Folic Acid.

Minerals: Calcium, Copper, Magnesium, Manganese, Phosphorus, Potassium, Silicon, Sodium, and Zinc.

Also: Coenzyme Q10, Protein, and Unsaturated fatty acids.

Helpful foods: Green leafy vegetables, nuts, oat bran, apples, apricots, bananas, citrus fruits, and seafood.

Juices: Beet greens, celery, green kale, and parsley juice.

PERNICIOUS ANEMIA

SPECIFICS: Pernicious anemia is caused from a deficiency of the vitamin B12, which in turn causes the gradual reduction in the number of blood cells, because the bone marrow is unable to produce mature red blood cells. This disease may be fatal without treatment. A highly nutritious diet, supplemented with large amounts of desiccated liver, and B12 injections are the recommended treatment.

(Beneficial Remedies, Treatments, and Nutrients)

Vitamins: B complex, B1, B2, B12, Folic acid, Niacin, C, and E.

Minerals: Cobalt, Copper, Iron, and Magnesium.

Also: Protein and L-Tryptophan.

Helpful foods: Apples, peaches, brewers yeast, citrus fruits, clams, eggs, kidney, soybeans, spinach, sweet potatoes, turnip greens, red meat, whole rye, and wheat.

Juices: Grape juice.

PERTUSSIS
(refer to Whooping Cough - page 173)

PHLEBITIS

SPECIFICS: An Inflammation of the vein wall (usually found in the legs) and can be a complication of varicose veins. Prevention and treatment require a diet rich in vitamins B, C, and E, plus regular exercise.

(Beneficial Remedies, Treatments, and Nutrients)

HERBAL COMBINATIONS: (H Formula) (Garlicin HC).

PHYSIOLOGIC ACTION: The herbs in these combinations are known to strengthen and support the cardiovascular system. Supplementing the body with niacin (B3) may be useful to help prevent clot formation. Vitamin C can help strengthen the blood vessel walls. Some research indicates that vitamin E may dilate the blood vessels, thus discouraging the formation of varicose veins and phlebitis.

Single herbs: Ginkgo, Horse Chestnut, and Yarrow.

Vitamins: B complex, Niacin, Pantothenic acid, C, and E.

Minerals: A multi-mineral complex.

Helpful foods: Beef, broccoli, fruit(citrus and other), nuts, green leafy vegetables, turnip greens, vegetable oils, and unpolished rice.

PILES
(refer to Hemorrhoids - page 83)

PINK EYE

SPECIFICS: A highly contagious inflammation of the mucous membrane that lines the eyelids. The most common cause of pink eye is a calcium deficiency, however allergies, bacteria, and a deficiency of vitamin A, B6, or riboflavin may cause pink eye symptoms.

(Beneficial Remedies, Treatments, and Nutrients)

Single herbs: Hot compresses made from Chamomile or Fennel tea may be helpful for irritation.

Vitamins: A, B2, B6, B complex, Niacin, C, and D.

Minerals: Calcium, Magnesium, Phosphorus, and Zinc.

Helpful foods: Apricots, citrus fruits, cherries, beef, black molasses, broccoli, carrots, butter, cheese, shell fish, tuna, and whole wheat.

PINWORMS
(refer to Parasites - page 126)

PLEURITIS

SPECIFICS: A type of skin eruption characterized by tiny blisters that weep and crust. Chronic forms produce flaking, scaling, itching, and eventual thickening and color changes of the skin.

(Beneficial Remedies, Treatments, and Nutrients)

HERBAL COMBINATION: (AKN).

PHYSIOLOGIC ACTION: When toxins are not properly eliminated from the body, they may surface through the skin creating pleuritis. This formula has been created to support liver and gall bladder function, to ensure toxins are filtered from the blood.

Single herbs: Aloe Vera, Chickweed, Evening Primrose Oil, Pau d'Arco, Red Clover, Thisilyn (Milk Thistle), and Yellow Dock.

Vitamins: A, B2, B3, B5, B6, C, F, P, Biotin, and Paba.

Minerals: Iron, Silicon, and Sulfur.

Also: Yu-ccan herbal drink, Whey powder, and Brewers yeast.

Helpful foods: Almonds, avocados, apricots, citrus fruits, red meat, seafood's, broccoli, carrots, radish, sweet potatoes, turnip greens, and fish liver oils.

PNEUMONIA

SPECIFICS: An inflammation in the lungs, characterized by the tiny air sacs in the lung area becoming inflamed and filled with mucus and pus. The primary causes of pneumonia are allergies, bacteria, chemical irritants, and viruses.

(Beneficial Remedies, Treatments, and Nutrients)

HERBAL COMBINATIONS: (Garlicin) (C+F) (Herbal Influence).

PHYSIOLOGIC ACTION: Proven herbal formulas to help relieve symptoms of colds, flu, hoarseness, colic, cramps, sluggish circulation, beginning of fevers, and germinal viral infections.

Herbal Influence (formerly known as Herbal Composition) was created by the early American herbalist, Samuel Thomson. It contains herbs which help with fever and nauseousness.

Single herbs: Boneset, Comfrey, EchinaGuard, Eucalyptus, Fenugreek, Licorice, & Mullein.

Vitamins: A, B complex, Ester C with Bioflavonoids, E, K, and P.

Minerals: Zinc.

Also: Coenzyme Q10, Germanium, L-Carnitine, L-Cysteine, Proteolytic enzymes, and Raw thymus extract.

Helpful foods: Apricots, citrus fruits, buckwheat, soybeans, nuts, broccoli, carrots, green leafy vegetables, garlic, kelp, herring, and oysters.

Juices: Aloe Vera juice.

POISON IVY

SPECIFICS: If the sap of the poison ivy touches the skin, it can cause persistent itching, rash, swelling, and blistering in sensitive people. The following nutrients will help alleviate the symptoms.

(Beneficial Remedies, Treatments, and Nutrients)

Single herbs: Echinacea, Goldenseal, and Lobelia.

Vitamins: A, C, and E.

Minerals: Zinc.

Helpful foods: Broccoli, carrots, citrus fruits, melon, fish liver oils, and vegetable oils.

POLIO

SPECIFICS: Polio is a virus infection of the spinal cord, which destroys the nerves controlling muscular movement. During the infectious stage, the rapid tissue destruction causes a depletion of protein and potassium.

(Beneficial Remedies, Treatments, and Nutrients)

Vitamins: A, B complex, and C.

Minerals: Calcium, Magnesium, Potassium, and Sodium.

Also: Protein.

Helpful foods: Bacon, beef, chicken, cheese and other dairy products, eggs, seafood's, apples, bananas, citrus fruits, peanuts, and unpolished rice.

POLYMYALGIA RHEUMATICA

SPECIFICS: This disorder causes pain in the joints, stiffness of muscles, and minor aches and twinges

(Beneficial Remedies, Treatments, and Nutrients)

HERBAL COMBINATIONS: (Yucca-AR) or (Rheum-Aid).

PHYSIOLOGIC ACTION: Excellent formulas for relieving symptoms associated with polymyalgia rheumatica. It helps to reduce or eliminate swelling, inflammation in joints, connective tissues, and relieves stiffness and pain.

Single herbs: Alfalfa, Chaparral, Cayenne, Fennel, Garlic, Pau d'Arco, Red Clover, Red Raspberry, and Yucca.

HOMEOPATHIC COMBINATION: Arthritis Pain Formula.

Vitamins: B complex, B5, B15, C, and E.

Minerals: Calcium, Magnesium, Phosphorus, Potassium, and Zinc.

Also: Digestive enzymes, Yu-ccan herbal drink, Hydrochloric acid, and Protein.

Helpful foods: Almonds, apricots, beef, butter, broccoli, buckwheat, all fruits, cheese, sardines, soybeans, spinach, safflower, goats milk, and mung beans.

POLYPS

SPECIFICS: Benign growths found on the epithelial lining of the cervix, bladder, or large intestine.

(Beneficial Remedies, Treatments, and Nutrients)

Single herbs: Pau d'Arco.

Vitamins: Multi-vitamin complex plus A, C, and E.

Minerals: Calcium.

Also: Aerobic bulk cleanse, Coenzyme Q10, and Germanium.

Helpful foods: Carrots, citrus fruits, melon, oat bran, soybeans, green leafy vegetables, vegetable oils, dairy products, and garlic.

POOR CIRCULATION

SPECIFICS: There are many disorders associated with circulatory problems. The most common disease for sluggish circulation is Raynaud's Disease, characterized by constriction and spasm of the blood vessels in the limbs. Poor circulation can also result from varicose veins, caused by the loss of elasticity in the walls of the veins.

(Beneficial Remedies, Treatments, and Nutrients)

HERBAL COMBINATIONS: (H Formula) (Ginkgold).

PHYSIOLOGIC ACTION: Contains herbs which strengthen the heart and build the vascular system. When taken with Cayenne, it improves circulation, giving a warming sensation to the entire body.

Note: Cayenne strengthens the pulse rate and circulation, while Black Cohosh slows it down.

Single herbs: Cayenne, Black Cohosh, Bayberry, Butchers Broom, Ginkgo, Hawthorn berries, Horsetail, Rose Hips, and Yarrow.

Vitamins: A, B complex, B1, B3, B6, B12, C, and E.

Minerals: Calcium, Magnesium, Potassium, and Zinc.

Also: Chlorophyll, Coenzyme Q10, Germanium, Lecithin, L-Carnitine, and Multidigestive enzymes.

Helpful foods: Apples, lean beef, broccoli, fruits(citrus and other),sprouted seeds, sunflower seeds, sweet potatoes, sardines, tuna, turnip greens, and yellow corn.

Juices: Alfalfa, blackberry, beetroot, parsley, and pineapple juice.

POSTURAL HYPOTENSION
(refer to Blood Pressure Low - page 25)

PREMENSTRUAL SYNDROME
(PMS)

SPECIFICS: A disorder that effects menstruating women before the menstrual cycle begins. The most common causes are candidiasis, food allergies, hormone imbalance, fluid retention, and low blood sugar. Symptoms can include one or all of the following; depression, cramps, headache, changes in personality, nervousness, fatigue, insomnia, breast swelling, and bloated abdomen. The best prevention for PMS is a nutrient rich diet, supplemented with vitamins and minerals, plus a good exercise program.

(Beneficial Remedies, Treatments, and Nutrients)

HERBAL COMBINATIONS: (FC) or (FEM-MEND).

PHYSIOLOGIC ACTION: Helps regulate the menstrual cycle, re-lieve cramps, bloating and vaginitis, ease inflammation of the vagina and uterus, and strengthen and regulate the kidneys, bladder and uterus areas. Beneficial for all female and uterine complaints.

WARNING: Do not use this combination while taking estrogen or oral contraceptives!

Single herbs: Dong Quai, Kelp, Red Raspberry, and Uva Ursi.

HOMEOPATHIC COMBINATION: PMS Formula.

Vitamins: B complex, B5, B6, B12, C, D, and E.

Minerals: Calcium, Chlorine, Chromium, Iodine, Iron, Magnesium, and Manganese.

Also: Inositol, L-Lysine, L-Tyrosine, Methionine, Spirulina, and Primrose oil.

Helpful foods: All vegetables and vegetable oils, fish and fish liver oils, cheese, butter, apples, bananas, citrus fruits, and mushrooms.

PRE-NATAL PREPARATION

SPECIFICS: Pre-natal preparation includes involves regular tests on the woman and the fetus to detect defects, disease, or potential hazards, and advising the woman on the general aspects of pregnancy , such as a well balanced diet and exercise, with the aim of making sure that the baby and mother are healthy at delivery.

(Beneficial Remedies, Treatments, and Nutrients)

HERBAL COMBINATION: (Healthy Greens).

PHYSIOLOGIC ACTION: A complete combination of vitamins and minerals containing digestive aids to ensure proper assimilation.

Single herbs: Blessed Thistle, Chamomile, Chlorella, Lobelia, and Red Raspberry.

Vitamins: A, B complex, B12, C, D, and E.

Minerals: A multi-mineral complex, plus Calcium, Magnesium, and Phosphorus.

Also: Bone meal, brewer's yeast, and kelp.

Helpful foods: All fruits (citrus and other), all dairy products, carrots, corn, soybeans, spinach, sprouted seeds, sweet potatoes, nuts, tuna, and red meat.

PRESBYOPIA

SPECIFICS: Presbyopia is one of the leading causes of decreased visual acuity in the elderly. This condition is characterized by the eye lens becoming less flexible.

Poor nutrition will accelerate the deterioration of your eyes. Improved nutrition will not reverse the condition but it will slow the progress of this ailment. Consumption of saturated fats, white sugar, and refined carbohydrates should be avoided.

(Beneficial Remedies, Treatments, and Nutrients)

Single herbs: Gingko Biloba, Bilberry, and Hawthorn.

Vitamins: A, Beta-carotene, C, and E.

Minerals: Selenium and Zinc.

Also: Bioflavonoids, Omega-3, and Omega-6.

Helpful foods: Broccoli, carrots, citrus fruits, garlic, strawberries, vegetable oils, and fish liver oils.

PROLAPSUS

SPECIFICS: The displacement of all or part of an organ or tissue from its normal position. This condition is caused by weakening and slackness of the various muscles, ligaments, and connective tissues.

(Beneficial Remedies, Treatments, and Nutrients)

HERBAL COMBINATION: (Yellow dock Combination).

PHYSIOLOGIC ACTION: Helps revitalize a prolapsed uterus, kidneys, and bowel. It also has been proven effective for hemorrhoids, colitis, and as a good purifier.

Single herbs: Black Walnut hull, Calendula flower, Marshmallow root, Mullein, White Oak bark, and Yellow Dock root.

Helpful foods: Beet root, black cherry, carrot, celery, cucumber, and radish juice.

PROSTATE and KIDNEY DISORDERS

SPECIFICS: Prostatitis is the inflammation of the prostrate gland, that is usually caused in older males by a gradual enlargement over a period of years, and in younger men by a bacterial infection from another area of the body, which has invaded the prostate. Prostatitis can partially or totally block the flow of urine, resulting in urine retention. Symptoms of prostatitis are fever, frequent urination accompanied by a burning sensation, pain between the scrotum and rectum, and blood or pus in the urine.

Treatment consists of regularity in sexual habits, the following nutrients, and lots of walking and other exercise.

(Beneficial Remedies, Treatments, and Nutrients)

HERBAL COMBINATION: (PR).

PHYSIOLOGIC ACTION: This formula helps cleanse sedimentation and arrest infection in the prostate and dissolve kidney stones to restore these glands to the natural functions.

Single herbs: Cayenne, Bee Pollen, Garlic, Golden Seal, Juniper Berries, Siberian Ginseng, and Uva Ursi.

Note: ProActive is an herbal extract of Saw Palmetto.

Vitamins: A, B complex, B6, C, E, and F.

Minerals: Calcium, Magnesium, and Zinc.

Also: Bee pollen, Brewer's yeast, Essential fatty acids, Lecithin, and Pumpkin seeds.

Helpful foods: All vegetables, apples, bananas, broccoli, carrots, cheese and other dairy products, tuna, and fish liver oils, red meat, and sprouted seeds.

Juices: Black currant, celery, and pomegranate juice.

PRURITUS ANI

SPECIFICS: A form of contact dermatitis, characterized by a burning sensation and itching of the rectum. Pruritus is associated with a deficiency of vitamins A, B complex, and Iron.

(Beneficial Remedies, Treatments, and Nutrients)

Single herbs: Kelp.

Vitamins: A and B complex.

Minerals: Iron.

Also: Acidophilus.

Helpful foods: Black molasses, brewers yeast, fish liver oils, vegetable oils, and red meat.

PSORIASIS

SPECIFICS: A hereditary disease that appears as patches of silvery scales or red areas on limbs, ears, and back. Attacks are triggered by inadequate diet, illness, viral and bacterial infection, sunburn, nervous tension, and stress.

Since diet and stress are key factors in this skin disorder, certain allergen foods need to be completely avoided. Dairy products and wheat are especially harmful in many instances. Fat should be kept to a minimum.

(Beneficial Remedies, Treatments, and Nutrients)

HERBAL COMBINATIONS: (AKN) (Evening Primrose) (Thisilyn).

PHYSIOLOGIC ACTION: The above herbs taken in combination has a dramatic effect on this disorder.

Single herbs: Chickweed, Dandelion, Goldenseal, Kelp, Lobelia, Skullcap, St. Johns Wort, and Yellow dock.

Vitamins: A, B5, B6, B12, B complex, C, D, E, and Folic Acid.

Minerals: Calcium, Magnesium, Sulfur ointment, and Zinc.

Also: Lecithin, Lipotropic factors, Proteolytic enzymes, and Unsaturated fatty acids.

Helpful foods: Apples, apricots, cherries, grapes, citrus fruits, all vegetables, beef, chicken, herring, oysters, tuna, salmon, and sardines.

EDEMA

SPECIFICS: Pulmonary edema is a fluid accumulation in the lungs. This ailment is usually caused left-sided heart failure, which results a in back-pressure of fluid in the lungs. Pulmonary edema may also be caused by allergies, chest infection, inhalation of irritant gases, or to any of the causes of generalized edema.

(Beneficial Remedies, Treatments, and Nutrients)

HERBAL COMBINATION: (KB).

PHYSIOLOGIC ACTION: KB acts as a mild diuretic to rid the lungs of excessive water.

Single herbs: Alfalfa, Buchu, Dandelion tea, Juniper, lobelia, Parsley, Pau d'Arco tea, Safflower, Uva Ursi, and Yarrow.

Vitamins: B1, B6, B complex, C, D, and E.

Minerals: Calcium, Copper, and Potassium.

Also: L-Taurine, #9 and #11 tissue salts, Silicon, low Sodium, and Protein.

Helpful foods: Fruit(citrus and other), beef, butter, cheese, egg whites, seafood, fish liver oils, broccoli, spinach, flax seed, and sunflower seeds.

PYORRHEA

SPECIFICS: An infectious disease of the gums and tooth sockets. This disease is characterized by the loosening of the teeth, the formation of pus, and tender or sore gums.

(Beneficial Remedies, Treatments, and Nutrients)

Single herbs: Golden Seal and Myrrh.

PHYSIOLOGIC ACTION: Use these powders on tooth brush, or make a tea, which is one teaspoon of each the Golden Seal and Myrrh, in one pint of boiling water. Steep. Rinse mouth and gargle with it freely, also, brush gums with the tea.

Vitamins: A, B complex, B1, B2, B6, B12, C, D, and E.

Minerals: Calcium, Magnesium, and Zinc.

Also: Protein. Also rub the gums, morning and evening, with vitamin E.

Helpful foods: Apples, citrus fruits, broccoli, carrots, green leafy vegetables, soybeans, sprouted seeds, seafood, red meat, and fish liver oils.

QUINSY

SPECIFICS: An abscess around the tonsil occurring as a complication of tonsillitis. The most effective prevention and treatment for tonsillitis and quinsy is a proper diet, high in vitamins, minerals, and protein.

(Beneficial Remedies, Treatments, and Nutrients)

HERBAL COMBINATION: (IF) (IGL).

PHYSIOLOGIC ACTION: Effective formulas that help cleanse toxins, combat infections, and reduce infection. Especially effective for healing the lymphatic system.

Single herbs: Bayberry Root, Echina Guard, Echinacea, Ginger Root and Pau d'Arco.

Vitamins and Minerals: A complete, one a day multi complex.

Also: Canaid herbal drink.

Helpful foods: Beef, broccoli, fruit(citrus and other), nuts, soybeans, spinach, sweet potatoes, turnip greens, unpolished rice, and whole grains.

RAYNAUD'S DISEASE

SPECIFICS: The most common disease for sluggish circulation is Raynaud's disease, characterized by constriction and spasm of the blood vessels in the limbs, resulting in hands and feet that are hypersensitive to the cold.

(Beneficial Remedies, Treatments, and Nutrients)

HERBAL COMBINATIONS: (H Formula) (Ginkgold).

PHYSIOLOGIC ACTION: Contains herbs which strengthen the heart and build the vascular system. When taken with Cayenne, it improves circulation, giving a warming sensation to the entire body.

Single herbs: Cayenne, Bayberry, Butchers Broom, Garlic, Ginkgo Biloba, Pau d'Arco, and Yarrow.

Vitamins: A, B3, B6, C, and E.

Minerals: Calcium, Magnesium, and Potassium.

Also: Chlorophyll, Coenzyme Q10, Germanium, and Lecithin.

Helpful foods: Brewers yeast, broccoli, carrots, kelp, soybeans, sunflower seeds, white meat of poultry, and vegetable oils.

RENAL CALCULI
(refer to Kidney and Bladder Stones - page 97)

RESTLESS LEG SYNDROME

SPECIFICS: Characterized by unpleasant burning, prickling, tickling, or aching sensations in the muscles of the legs. Symptoms are most common during prolonged sitting or at night in bed. This ailment is most likely to occur in individuals that who consume large amounts of coffee, heavy smokers, and people with rheumatoid arthritis.

(Beneficial Remedies, Treatments, and Nutrients)

Single herbs: Alfalfa, Black Cohosh, Burdock, Cayenne, Celery seed, Chaparral, Devil's Claw, Valerian root, and Yucca.

HOMEOPATHIC COMBINATION: Arthritis Pain Formula.

Vitamins: Niacin, B5, B6, B12, B complex, C, E, and Folic acid.

Minerals: A strong Multi-mineral complex, plus Calcium, Magnesium, and Potassium.

Also: Cod liver oil, Green Magma, Aqua life, Seatone, and Omega-3 oils..

Helpful foods: Almonds, apricots, beef, butter, broccoli, buckwheat, all fruits, cheese, sardines, soybeans, spinach, sprouts, safflower, goats milk, and peanuts.

Juices: Parsley and celery juice; cherry and pineapple juice.

RHEUMATIC FEVER

SPECIFICS: Rheumatic fever is an infection, caused by streptococcal bacteria. It most often effects children aged three to eighteen. A salt restricted diet, containing bioflavonoids and all essential nutrients has been found valuable for treating and preventing rheumatic fever.

(Beneficial Remedies, Treatments, and Nutrients)

Single herbs: Birch leaves, Catnip, Dandelion, Fenugreek, Garlic, Lobelia, and Thyme.

Vitamins: A, B2, B6, B complex C, D, and E.

Minerals: Zinc.

Also: Bioflavonoids, Coenzyme Q10, Germanium, Primadophilus, Protein, and Proteolytic enzymes.

Helpful foods: Beef, chicken, oysters, herring, tuna, carrots, green leafy vegetables, fruit(citrus and other), soybeans, sprouted seeds, and whole wheat.

Juices: Aloe Vera and citrus juices.

RHEUMATISM

SPECIFICS: Rheumatism is a general term referring to pain in the joints and stiffness of muscles.

(Beneficial Remedies, Treatments, and Nutrients)

HERBAL COMBINATIONS: (Yucca-AR) or (Rheum-Aid).

PHYSIOLOGIC ACTION: Excellent formulas for relieving symptoms associated with bursitis, calcification, gout, rheumatoid arthritis, rheumatism, and osteoarthritis. It helps to reduce or eliminate swelling, inflammation in joints, connective tissues, and relieves stiffness and pain.

Single herbs: Alfalfa, Chaparral, Cayenne, Fennel, Garlic, Pau d'Arco, Red Clover, Red Raspberry, and Yucca.

HOMEOPATHIC COMBINATION: Arthritis Pain Formula.

Vitamins: B complex, B5, B15, C, and E.

Minerals: Calcium, Magnesium, Phosphorus, Potassium, and Zinc.

Also: Digestive enzymes, Yu-ccan herbal drink, Hydrochloric acid, and Protein.

Helpful foods: Almonds, apricots, beef, butter, broccoli, buckwheat, all fruits, cheese, sardines, soybeans, spinach, safflower, goats milk, and mung beans.

Juices: Cucumber, parsley and celery juice; cherry and pineapple juice.

RICKETS

SPECIFICS: A disease of malnutrition caused by a deficiency of calcium, phosphorus, and vitamin D. This causes the bones to become soft, resulting in deformities.

(Beneficial Remedies, Treatments, and Nutrients)

Single herbs: Horsetail.

Vitamins: A, B12, C, and D.

Minerals: Calcium, Magnesium, and Phosphorus.

Also: Cod liver oil, Lecithin, Hydrochloric acid, Silica, and Digestive enzymes.

Helpful foods: Apples, citrus fruits, melon, cheese and other dairy products, beef, chicken, seafood's, all vegetables, nuts, and sunflower seeds.

Juices: Dandelion and orange juice.

RINGING IN EARS
(refer to Tinnitus - page 161)

RINGWORM

SPECIFICS: A highly contagious, yeast-like, fungal infection, that lives off dead skin cells. Ring worm victims should eat a well-balanced diet, supplemented by megadoses of vitamins A, B, and C.

(Beneficial Remedies, Treatments, and Nutrients)

HERBAL COMBINATION: (Black Walnut extract).

PHYSIOLOGIC ACTION: High in organic iodine, this herb has proven effective against fungal infections such as ringworm and athletes foot.

Single herbs: Black Walnut, Golden Seal, and Pau d'Arco.

Vitamins: A, B complex, and C.

Minerals: Zinc.

Also: Acidophilus, Caprinex (caprylic acid), Germanium, and Unsaturated fatty acids. Rub skin with Black Walnut extract, Apple Cider Vinegar or Castor Oil, several times a day.

Helpful foods: Egg yolk, apricot, citrus fruits, beef kidney, beef liver, vegetable and fish oils.

ROUNDWORMS

SPECIFICS: Roundworms live in the gastrointestinal tract. Early signs include diarrhea, loss of appetite, and rectal itching. If not eliminated they will result in the loss of weight, colon disorders, and anemia. Causes include ingestion of eggs or larvae from partially cooked meat, improper disposal of human waste, and walking barefoot on contaminated soil.

(Beneficial Remedies, Treatments, and Nutrients)

HERBAL COMBINATIONS: (Para-X) (Para-VF).

PHYSIOLOGIC ACTION: Useful in destroying and eliminating parasites, such as worms. Also helps relieve many kinds of skin problems. The Para-VF is a liquid and is useful for children and the elderly who cannot swallow capsules.

Warning: Do not use during pregnancy!

Single herbs: Black Walnut, Garlic, Pumpkin Seeds, Sage, Sheep Sorrel, Swedish Bitters and Wormwood.

Vitamins: Folic Acid.

Minerals: Multi-mineral complex.

CHILDREN: Chamomile tea or raisins soaked in Senna tea, for older children, may be helpful.

Helpful foods: Asparagus, brewers yeast, broccoli, lettuce, lima beans, liver, mushrooms, nuts, and spinach.

RUBELLA
(refer to Measles - page 106)

SCARS
(refer to Skin Problems - page 149)

SCIATICA

SPECIFICS: Sciatica refers to painful spasms along the sciatic nerve which runs from the back of the thigh, down the inside of the leg to the ankle. Causes of sciatica are ruptured discs or sprained joints in the lower back, inflammation of sciatic nerve, or neuritis.

(Beneficial Remedies, Treatments, and Nutrients)

Single herbs: Pau d'Arco.

Vitamins: B1, B12, B complex, D, and E.

Minerals: Multi-mineral.

Helpful foods: Beef, tuna, butter, cheese, vegetable oils, sprouted seeds, soybeans, and sunflower seeds.

SCURVY

SPECIFICS: A malnutrition disease caused by vitamin D deficiency. A well-balanced diet, high in calcium, iron, protein, and vitamin D is recommended.

(Beneficial Remedies, Treatments, and Nutrients)

Single herbs: Kelp.

Vitamins: A, B complex, C, and D.

Minerals: Calcium, Iron, and Magnesium.

Also: Protein.

Helpful foods: Broccoli, carrots, green leafy vegetables, citrus fruits, apples, apricots, cherries, grapes, pineapple, and turnip greens.

SEBORRHEA

SPECIFICS: Seborrhea is a disorder of the glands that secrete oil (sebaceous glands). This disease is, nearly always, caused by a nutrient deficiency.

(Beneficial Remedies, Treatments, and Nutrients)

Single herbs: Chaparral, Dandelion, Goldenseal, and Red Clover.

Vitamins: A, B complex, B6, and E.

Minerals: Multi-mineral complex.

Also: Acidophilus, Coenzyme Q10, Lecithin, Protein supplement, and Unsaturated fatty acids.

Helpful foods: Carrots, green leafy vegetables, turnip greens, vegetable oils, fish liver oils, beef, all fruits, soybeans, nuts, and unpolished rice.
Juices: Carrot, tomato, and pineapple juice.

SEBORRHEIC DERMATITIS .

SPECIFICS: A red, scaly, itchy rash that develops on the back, chest, face, and chest.

(Beneficial Remedies, Treatments, and Nutrients)

HERBAL COMBINATION: (AKN).

PHYSIOLOGIC ACTION: Many skin problems are related to liver dysfunction. This formula gives support to the liver, helps to cleanse the blood, and supplies nutrients for the skin.

Single herbs: Aloe Vera (on skin), Burdock, Cleavers, Dandelion, Evening Primrose, Garlic, Golden Seal, Pau d'Arco, Yellowdock, and Yucca.

Vitamins: A, B complex, B2, B3, B6, D, E, and Biotin B complex.

Minerals: Sulfur ointment, Potassium, and Zinc.

Also: Yu-ccan herbal drink, and Protein.

SEIZURES
(refer to Epilepsy - page 63)

SENILITY

SPECIFICS: Senility occurs in old age and is usually caused by cerebral dysfunction, nervous disturbances, and strokes.

(Beneficial Remedies, Treatments, and Nutrients)

HERBAL COMBINATIONS: (SEN) or (Remem).

PHYSIOLOGIC ACTION: An excellent combination to nourish the brain cells and tissues. Improves their ability to perform mental functions.

Note: Often a nutritional deficiency is the cause.

Single herbs: Dandelion, Ginkgo, Ginseng, Gotu Kola, Licorice, and Yellow Dock.

Vitamins: A, B3, B complex, C, and E.

Minerals: Choline and Zinc.

Also: Coenzyme Q10, Germanium, Lecithin, and Protein.

Helpful foods: Aloe Vera, avocados, citrus fruits, broccoli, carrots, garlic, olives, soybeans, spinach, sweet potatoes, whole wheat, oat bran, herring, and oysters.

Juices: Carrot, celery, and prune juice.

<u>SHINGLES</u> (Herpes Zoster)

SPECIFICS: Shingles is an infection caused by a virus of the nerve endings in the skin. It usually occurs on the skin of the abdomen under the ribs. If shingles develop near the eyes, the cornea may become affected, causing blindness. B vitamins are necessary for the proper functioning of the nerves. Vitamins A and C promote healing of skin lesions and heavy doses of vitamin C can limit infection of lesions.

(Beneficial Remedies, Treatments, and Nutrients)

Single herbs: Yucca.

Vitamins: A, B1, B6, B12, B complex, C, and D.

Minerals: Calcium and Magnesium.

Also: L-Lysine and Protein.

Helpful foods: Red meat, butter, cheese, fruit(citrus and other), vegetable oils, nuts, sprouted seeds, and tuna.

<u>SICKLE - CELL ANEMIA</u>

SPECIFICS: Sickle-cell anemia is caused from a deficiency of folic acid, which in turn causes the red blood cells to become bent (sickled) and hard, clogging the circulatory system, depriving the body tissues of oxygen. The recommended treatment is a highly nutritious diet, supplemented with large amounts of desiccated liver, vitamin C, and folic acid.

(Beneficial Remedies, Treatments, and Nutrients)

Vitamins: B complex, B1, B2, B12, Folic acid, Niacin, C, and E.

Minerals: Cobalt, Copper, Iron, and Magnesium.

Also: Protein and L-Tryptophan.

Helpful foods: Citrus fruits, apples, red meat, clams, kidney, soybeans, spinach, sweet potatoes, whole wheat, and whole rye.

Juices: Asparagus, lettuce, lima beans, spinach, and deep green vegetable juices.

SINUSITIS

SPECIFICS: Sinusitis is an inflammation of one or more of the nasal sinus cavities, that accompanies upper respiratory infection. Sinusitis may be the result of colds or viral and bacterial infections of the nose, throat, and upper respiratory tract.

(Beneficial Remedies, Treatments, and Nutrients)

HERBAL COMBINATIONS: (HAS) (Zand Decongest Herbal Formula) (Garlicin CF) (Fenu-Thyme) (Sinustop).

PHYSIOLOGIC ACTION: Promote sinus drainage and shrink swollen membranes. The above are all recommended natural sinus decongestants that help relieve nasal congestion and pressure associated with sinusitis.

Single herbs: Anis, Comfrey, Elderberry, Eyebright, Fenugreek, Golden Seal, Horehound, Lobelia, Marshmallow, Mullein, Red Clover, and Rose Hips.

HOMEOPATHIC COMBINATION: Sinusitis Formula.

Vitamins: A, B complex, B5, C, and E.

Minerals: Potassium and Zinc.

Also: Bee Pollen, Coenzyme Q10, Garlic capsules, Germanium, Protein, and Proteolytic enzymes.

Helpful foods: Apples, citrus fruit, celery, herring, oysters, and turnip greens.

Juices: Lemon juice with a little horseradish.

SKIN *(Bites, Stings, and Poisons)*

SPECIFICS: More people die from bee stings than from poisonous bites. People with known allergies to bites or stings should carry vitamin C with them; if bitten take large amounts of C immediately and frequently thereafter.

(Beneficial Remedies, Treatments, and Nutrients)

HERBAL COMBINATION: (EchinaGuard).

PHYSIOLOGIC ACTION: Echinacea was used by the Plains Indians to lessen the effects of poisonous bites. EchinaGuard would be very beneficial. Take large doses of vitamin C and Calcium. Use vitamin E topically to reduce pain.

Single herbs: Echinacea.

Vitamins: Multi-vitamin complex.

Minerals: Mineral complex.

Helpful foods: Broccoli, cauliflower, tomatoes, dark leafy vegetables, apples, black currants, citrus fruits, almonds, sesame seeds, sardines, and salmon.

SKIN *(Acne, Pimples, etc.)*

SPECIFICS: A disorder of the oil(sebaceous) glands in the skin. It is believed that stress is a significant factor in acne. Other factors that contribute to acne and pimples are allergies, heredity, oral contraceptives, overindulgence in carbohydrates, foods with high fat or sugar content, and androgens(male hormones) produced in increased amounts when the girl or boy reaches puberty.

(Beneficial Remedies, Treatments, and Nutrients)

Single herbs: Hautex, and Yucca.

PHYSIOLOGIC ACTION: The above herbs work from within to encourage skin secretion, effective for acne, blackheads, pimples, itch, and rash.

Vitamins: A, B complex, E, and C with Rosehips.

Minerals: Calcium and Zinc.

Also: Yu-ccan herbal drink, Efamol, Whey Powder, and Acidophilus.

Helpful foods: Avocados, bananas, broccoli, lean beef, carrots, celery, fruits (citrus and other), green leafy vegetables, pumpkin, radish, and vegetable oils.

SKIN BLEMISHES

SPECIFICS: A small circumscribed alteration of the skin considered to be unesthetic but insignificant.

(Beneficial Remedies, Treatments, and Nutrients)

HERBAL COMBINATION: (AKN).

PHYSIOLOGIC ACTION: AKN helps cleanse the bloodstream. Pimples, blackheads, and other superficial skin eruptions, and more serious conditions such as boils, carbuncles, dermatitis, eczema, and pleuritis will be eliminated when the blood has been cleansed.

Vitamins: A, B2, B3, B5, B6, C, F, P, Biotin, and Paba.

Minerals: Iron, Silicon, and Sulfur.

Also: Whey Powder and Brewers Yeast.

Helpful foods: Almonds, apricots, avocados, citrus fruits, fish liver oils, carrots, radish, sweet potatoes, green leafy vegetables, vegetable oils, and flax seed.

SKIN CANCER
(refer to Melanoma - page 107)

SKIN PROBLEMS
(Beneficial Remedies, Treatments, and Nutrients)

Age Spots - B complex, B5, C, Lactobacillus bulgaricus.

Dry Skin — Chamomile, Dandelion, Lavender, Peppermint, Oat Extract, Evening Primrose Oil, Vitamin A, B complex, C, and Aloe Vera. Add Herbal oils to bath (Lavender oil is very nice).

Itchy Skin — Chickweed, Calendula, Elder, Yarrow, vegetable oil daily, and apple cider vinegar to bath. X-Itch ointment is also very effective.

Oily Skin — Vitamin B complex, Liver, Lemon Grass, Licorice root, Rosemary, and Rose buds.

Scars — Vitamin E orally and topically.

Stretch marks — Vitamin E, B complex, B5, C, Aloe Vera, Zinc, and Carnation oil.

Sunburn — B vitamins, Paba, C, E, Calcium, Zinc, and Aloe Vera.

Wrinkles — Vitamins A, B complex, E, Zinc, Selenium, and Almond oil.

SMOKING

SPECIFICS: Tobacco smoke contains over 3,700 compounds, most are toxic and many are carcinogenic. 90% of lung cancer is due to smoking and over 30% of all cancer deaths can be attributed to smoking. The risk of developing lung cancer begins to deminish as soon as smoking is stopped.

(Beneficial Remedies, Treatments, and Nutrients)

HERBAL COMBINATIONS: (Milk thistle extract) or (Thisilyn).

PHYSIOLOGIC ACTION: The herbal combination decreases the desire for tobacco and protects the liver from the negative effects of smoking. Vitamins and minerals should be taken to rebuild the nutritional system after a juice fast. The juice fast cleanses the accumulated poisons from the body, thus eliminating the physiological dependence.

Note: Tobacco, alcohol, caffeine, and other drug "cravings" are brought about by a physiological body dependence on the poison which develops during prolonged use. The addicts blood poison level must remain at a certain level at all times. As the poison level drops, there is a "desire" to take in more of the drug, to bring the level back again.

(Beneficial Remedies, Treatments, and Nutrients)

Single herbs: Catnip, Chaparral, Hops, Licorice, Lobelia, Skullcap, Slippery Elm, and Valerian.

Vitamins and Minerals: All.

Amino Acids: L- Cysteine, L- Cystine, and L- Methionine.

Also: Coenzyme Q10, Germanium, and Raw thymus.

Fasting: Drink juice only.

SNAKE BITE

SPECIFICS: All snake bite victims should remain as still as possible and should be seen by a doctor immediately. After seeing a doctor the following supplements will help alleviate pain and symptoms.

(Beneficial Remedies, Treatments, and Nutrients)

Single herbs: Echinacea, and Yellow dock.

Vitamins: B5, and C.

Minerals: Calcium.

Helpful foods: Brewers yeast, egg yolk, liver, rosehips, strawberries, and wheat germ.

SPASTIC COLON
(refer to Colitis - page 47)

SPIDER AND SCORPION BITE

SPECIFICS: Rattlesnake and black widow venom are almost the same so should be treated similarly. Rid the body of as much poison as possible by encouraging bleeding and see your doctor immediately. After seeing a doctor the following supplements will help alleviate pain and symptoms.

(Beneficial Remedies, Treatments, and Nutrients)

Single herbs: Echinacea and Yellow dock.

Vitamins: B5 and C.

Minerals: Calcium.

Also: Apply Comfrey or Plantain salve.

Helpful foods: Same as snake bite.

SPONDYLITIS

SPECIFICS: Inflammation of the joints between the vertebrae in the spine. usually caused by osteoasthritis or rheumatoid arthritis. In rare cases it is caused by a bacterial infection that has spread from another area of the body.

(Beneficial Remedies, Treatments, and Nutrients)

HERBAL COMBINATION: (Rheum-Aid) or (Yucca -AR).

PHYSIOLOGIC ACTION: Relieves symptoms associated with bursitis, calcification, gout, rheumatoid arthritis, rheumatism, and osteoarthritis. Helps the body reduce or eliminate swelling and inflammation in the joints and connective tissue and helps to relieve stiffness and pain.

Single herbs: Alfalfa, Black Cohosh, Burdock, Cayenne, Celery seed, Chaparral, Devil's Claw, Valerian root, and Yucca.

HOMEOPATHIC COMBINATION: Arthritis Pain Formula.

Vitamins: Niacin, B5, B6, B12, B complex, C, D, E, F, and P.

Minerals: A strong Multi-mineral complex, plus Calcium, and Magnesium.

Also: Cod liver oil, Yu-ccan herbal drink, Green Magma, Aqua life, Seatone, and Bromelain.

Helpful foods: Almonds, apricots, beef, butter, broccoli, buckwheat, all fruits, cheese, sardines, soybeans, spinach, safflower, goats milk, and mung beans.

Juices: Parsley and celery juice; cherry and pineapple juice.

SPRAIN

SPECIFICS: If a person stresses a muscle beyond its capability the ligament connecting the bone to the muscle may tear causing a sprain. A well-balanced diet that is high in protein and the following supplement program will help these injuries heal.

(Beneficial Remedies, Treatments, and Nutrients)

HERBAL COMBINATION: (B F + C)

PHYSIOLOGIC ACTION: A special formula to aid in healing processes for torn cartilage's and ligaments.

Single herbs: White Oak Bark, Comfrey Root, Black Walnut Hulls, Lobelia, Skullcap and Yucca.

HOMEOPATHIC COMBINATION: Injury and Backache Formula.

Vitamins: B complex, B5, B6, B12, C, and E.

Minerals: A complete multi-mineral one a day, (time released).

Also: Bee pollen, Coenzyme Q10, Germanium, L-Arginine, L-Carnitine, L-Lysine, Green-Lipped Mussel, Liver, Protein, Proteolytic enzymes, Silica, and Unsaturated fatty acids.

Helpful foods: Beef, fruits, nuts, unpolished rice, soybeans, spinach, vegetable oils, liver, and whole wheat.

STASIS ULCER
(refer to Leg Ulcers - page 99)

STRETCH MARKS
(refer to Skin Problems - page 149)

STRESS

SPECIFICS: The body can handle some stress, but long term stress causes the body to break down. Long term stress occurs when the situation that causes anxiety is not relieved. Find the cause and handle it constructively. People experiencing stress should maintain a well-balanced diet and replace the nutrients depleted during stress.

(Beneficial Remedies, Treatments, and Nutrients)

HERBAL COMBINATIONS: (Calm aid) (Ex stress) (Kalmin extract).

PHYSIOLOGIC ACTION: Special formulas for insomnia and stress related conditions. Relieve nervous tension, rebuilds nerve sheaths. Soothing and calming effect on the whole nervous system.

Single herbs: Black Cohosh Root, Cayenne, Lady's Slipper, Skullcap, Valerian Root, and Yucca.

Vitamins: A, all B's, C, D, E, Paba, Folic Acid, and Choline.

Minerals: Calcium, Chromium, Copper, Iron, Selenium, and Zinc.

Also: L-Tyrosine and Protein.

Helpful foods: Dulse, flax seed, sea salt, fruit(citrus and other), bacon, beef, chicken, all dairy products, all vegetables, mushrooms, and whole rye.

Juices: Carrot, celery, lettuce, tomato, and prune juice.

STROKE

SPECIFICS: When the blood supply is cut off to an area of brain cells, resulting in the death of the deprived cells. Emphasis should be placed on the reduction of being overweight, restricting sodium consumption, and reduce cholesterol intake. A sensible diet is of the upmost importance.

(Beneficial Remedies, Treatments, and Nutrients)

HERBAL COMBINATION: (Garlicin HC).

PHYSIOLOGIC ACTION: A combination of herbs which supports the cardiovascular system. Helps to strengthen the heart, while building and cleansing the arteries and veins.

SPECIFICS: Recent animal studies suggest that vitamin C deficiency could be involved in the causation of stroke. E.F.A.s (essential fatty acids) play a fundamental role in keeping cell membranes fluid and flexible.

Single herbs: Cayenne, Comfrey, Evening Primrose Oil, Fish Oil, Garlic, Golden Seal, and Rose Hips.

Vitamins: B complex, C, E, Niacin, Inositol, and Choline.

Minerals: Multi-mineral plus Calcium and Magnesium.

Also: (E.F.A.s) — Fish oils and cold pressed vegetable oils.

Helpful foods: Fruits(citrus and other), green leafy vegetables, turnip greens, tuna, herring, sardines, salmon, oysters, and shellfish.

SUBSTANCE ABUSE
(refer to Drug Dependency - page 58)

SUNBURN
(refer to Skin Problems - page 149)

SWOLLEN GLANDS

SPECIFICS: A term commonly used to describe the enlargement of any of the lymph glands. Swollen glands may indicate a localized infection or may be a symptom of a more serious disease such as cancer, chicken pox, leukemia, measles, mononucleosis, syphilis, or tuberculosis. Treatment includes a well-balanced diet with an increased intake of fluids, calories, and protein.

(Beneficial Remedies, Treatments, and Nutrients)

HERBAL COMBINATION: (IGL).

PHYSIOLOGIC ACTION: Combats infection and reduces inflammation from the body, especially the lymphatic system, ears, throat, lungs, breasts, and organs of the body.

Single herbs: Propolis, Golden Seal, Pau d'Arco, Saw Palmetto, and Echinacea.

Vitamins: A good multi-vitamin plus C.

Minerals: Multi-mineral complex.

Helpful foods: Aloe Vera, apples, bananas, broccoli, oat bran, carrots, citrus fruits, green leafy vegetables, soybeans, sweet potatoes, turnip greens, vegetable oils, lean red meat, and fish liver oils.

Juices: Celery juice.

SYPHILIS

SPECIFICS: Syphilis is caused by a bacterium called Treponema pallidum and is transmitted through physical contact such as kissing, as well as sexual intimacy. Complications of syphilis may result in blindness, brain damage, heart disease, hearing loss, and sterility. Penicillin or another antibiotic is the usual treatment. In addition to medical treatment, an afflicted person should maintain a high nutrient diet to help repair the tissue damage that has occurred.

(Beneficial Remedies, Treatments, and Nutrients)

Single herbs: Echinacea, Goldenseal, Pau d'Arco and Suma.

Vitamins: B complex and K.

Minerals: Zinc.

Also: Acidophilus, Coenzyme Q10, Germanium, and Protein.

Helpful foods: All red meats, fruits, aloe vera, kelp, herring, oysters, liver, nuts, and yogurt.

TAPEWORMS

SPECIFICS: Tapeworms live in the gastrointestinal tract. Early signs include diarrhea, loss of appetite, and rectal itching. If not eliminated they will result in the loss of weight, colon disorders, and anemia. Causes include ingestion of eggs or larvae from partially cooked meat and improper disposal of human waste.

(Beneficial Remedies, Treatments, and Nutrients)

HERBAL COMBINATIONS: (Para-X) (Para-VF).

PHYSIOLOGIC ACTION: Useful in destroying and eliminating parasites, such as worms. Also helps relieve many kinds of skin problems. The Para-VF is a liquid and is useful for children and the elderly who cannot swallow capsules.

WARNING: Do not use during pregnancy!

Single herbs: Black Walnut, Garlic, Pumpkin Seeds, Sage, Swedish Bitters, and Wormwood.

Vitamins: Folic Acid.

Minerals: Iron and Zinc.

CHILDREN: Chamomile tea or raisins soaked in Senna tea for older children may be helpful.

Helpful foods: Asparagus, brewers yeast, broccoli, lettuce, lima beans, liver, mushrooms, nuts, and spinach.

TEETH and GUM DISORDERS

SPECIFICS: Although cavities are a major dental disease, Periodontitis(a gum disease) accounts for the loss of more teeth than cavities. Periodontitis is an inflammation of the bones and gums that surround and support the teeth, caused by improper cleaning of teeth and gums, poorly fitting dentures, loose fillings, or an inadequate diet. (Also refer to pyorrhea).

(Beneficial Remedies, Treatments, and Nutrients)

Single herbs: Chamomile, Echinacea, Lobelia, Myrrh Gum, and White Oak Bark.

Vitamins: A, B complex, C, D, P, Niacin, and Folic Acid.

Minerals: Calcium, Copper, Magnesium, Manganese, Phosphorus, Potassium, Silicon, Sodium, and Zinc.

Also: Protein and Unsaturated fatty acids.

Toothache — Primrose oil or oil of cloves.

Stained or yellow teeth — brush with fresh strawberries.

Helpful foods: All dairy products, red meat, chicken, tuna, salmon, sardines, all vegetables, and vegetable oils.

Juices: Beet greens, celery, kale, and parsley juice.

TEETH GRINDING (Bruxism)

SPECIFICS: Bruxism can develop if the bite needs adjusting, the teeth are out of line, or the teeth become sensitive to heat and cold. However, the most common cause of bruxism is a deficiency of calcium or pantothenic acid.

(Beneficial Remedies, Treatments, and Nutrients)

Single herbs: Chamomile and Skullcap.

Vitamins: Multi-vitamins, pantothenic acid, B complex. Take tablets before bed for best results.

Also: Bonemeal or other Calcium supplement.

Helpful foods: Brewers yeast, cheese, milk, butter, egg yolk, almonds, walnuts, fish, wheat germ, and oat bran.

TEETHING

SPECIFICS: The following nutrients are to help your infant cope with the irritation and pain that is associated with teething.

(Beneficial Remedies, Treatments, and Nutrients)

Single herbs: Lobelia Extract, Aloe Vera Gel, or Peppermint Oil can be rubbed on the gums.

HOMEOPATHIC COMBINATION: Teething Formula.

Tissue salts: Combination "R."

Also: Teething Tablets from Hylands.

TEMPEROMANDIBULAR JOINT SYNDROME (TMJ)

SPECIFICS: TMJ syndrome is usually caused by spasm of the chewing muscles, as the result of clenching the teeth due to emotional stress. Symptoms include a dull aching facial pain, tenderness of the jaw, and headaches. A correct diet and proper supplements often solve the problem.

(Beneficial Remedies, Treatments, and Nutrients)

Single herbs: Hops, Passionflower, Skullcap and Valerian Root.

Vitamins: B complex, B5, B6, and C.

Minerals: Calcium and Magnesium.

Also: Coenzyme Q10 and L- Tyrosine.

Helpful foods: Green leafy vegetables, fruit, brown rice, soybeans, and whole grains.

TENNIS ELBOW

SPECIFICS: Tennis elbow is caused by inflammation of the tendon that attaches the extensor muscles. This condition results from constant overuse of muscles.

(Beneficial Remedies, Treatments, and Nutrients)

HERBAL COMBINATION: (B F + C)

PHYSIOLOGIC ACTION: A special formula to aid in healing processes for swelling and inflammation.

Single herbs: White Oak Bark, Comfrey Root, Black Walnut Hulls, Lobelia, Skullcap and Yucca.

HOMEOPATHIC COMBINATION: Injury and Backache Formula.

Vitamins: B complex, B5, B6, B12, C, and E.

Minerals: A complete multi-mineral one a day, (time released).

Also: Bee pollen, Coenzyme Q10, Germanium, L-Arginine, L-Carnitine, L-Lysine, Green-Lipped Mussel, Liver, Protein, Proteolytic enzymes, Silica, and Unsaturated fatty acids.

Helpful foods: Beef, fruits, nuts, unpolished rice, soybeans, spinach, vegetable oils, liver, and whole wheat.

TENSION

SPECIFICS: Tension is generally a direct result of stress. The body can handle some stress but long term stress causes the body to break down.

Long term stress occurs when the situation that causes anxiety is not relieved. Find the cause and handle it constructively. People experiencing stress should maintain a well-balanced diet and replace the nutrients depleted during stress.

(Beneficial Remedies, Treatments, and Nutrients)

HERBAL COMBINATIONS: (Calm-aid) or (Ex stress comb).

PHYSIOLOGIC ACTION: A proven formula that is soothing, strengthening, and healing to the whole nervous system to relieve nervous tension and rebuild the nerve sheaths. Excellent aid for insomnia, chronic nervousness, and stress-related conditions.

Single herbs: Evening Primrose Oil, Hops, Mistletoe, Skullcap, and Valerian.

Vitamins: B complex, B1, B2, B3, B5, B6, and C.

Minerals: Calcium, Iodine, Iron, Magnesium, Phosphorus, Potassium, Silicon, and Sodium.

Helpful foods: Dulse, flax seed, sea salt, fruit(citrus and other), bacon, beef, chicken, all dairy products, all vegetables, mushrooms, and whole rye.

Juices: Carrot, celery, and prune juice.

THREADWORMS

SPECIFICS: Thread worms live in the gastrointestinal tract. Early signs include diarrhea, loss of appetite, and rectal itching. If not eliminated they will result in the loss of weight, colon disorders, and anemia. Causes include ingestion of eggs or larvae from partially cooked meat, improper disposal of human waste, and walking barefoot on contaminated soil.

(Beneficial Remedies, Treatments, and Nutrients)

HERBAL COMBINATIONS: (Para-X) (Para-VF).

PHYSIOLOGIC ACTION: Useful in destroying and eliminating parasites, such as thread worms. Also helps relieve many kinds of skin problems. The Para-VF is liquid and is useful for children and the elderly who cannot swallow capsules.

WARNING: Do not use during pregnancy!

Single herbs: Black Walnut, Garlic, Pumpkin Seeds, Sage, Swedish Bitters, and Wormwood.

Vitamins: Folic Acid.

Minerals: A multi-mineral complex.

Children: Chamomile tea or raisins soaked in Senna tea for older children may be helpful.

Helpful foods: Asparagus, brewers yeast, broccoli, lettuce, lima beans, liver, mushrooms, nuts, and spinach.

THROMBOPHLEBITIS

SPECIFICS: An Inflammation of the vein, often accompanied by clot formation (usually found in the legs) and can be a complication of varicose veins. Prevention and treatment require a diet rich in vitamins B, C, and E, plus regular exercise.

(Beneficial Remedies, Treatments, and Nutrients)

HERBAL COMBINATIONS: (H Formula) (Garlicin HC).

PHYSIOLOGIC ACTION: The herbs in these combinations are known to strengthen and support the cardiovascular system. Supplementing the body with niacin (B3) may be useful to help prevent clot formation. Vitamin C can help strengthen the blood vessel walls. Some research indicates that vitamin E may dilate the blood vessels, thus discouraging the formation of varicose veins and phlebitis.

Single herbs: Ginkgo, Horse Chestnut, and Yarrow.

Vitamins: B complex, Niacin, Pantothenic acid, C, and E.

Minerals: A multi-mineral complex.

Helpful foods: Beef, broccoli, fruit(citrus and other), nuts, green leafy vegetables, turnip greens, vegetable oils, and unpolished rice.

THROMBOSIS

SPECIFICS: Thrombosis is due to the gradual build-up of calcium and cholesterol-containing masses known as plaques on the inside of the artery walls. The clot will slow or restrict the circulation of the blood causing high blood pressure. Symptoms of this disease are cramping of muscles, chest pains and pressure, and hypertension. The main causes are poor diet, drug abuse, alcoholism, smoking, heredity, obesity, and stress.

(Beneficial Remedies, Treatments, and Nutrients)

HERBAL COMBINATION: (Garlicin HC).

PHYSIOLOGIC ACTION: A combination of herbs which supports the cardiovascular system. Helps to strengthen the heart, while building and cleansing the arteries and veins.

SPECIFICS: Recent animal studies suggest that vitamin C deficiency could be involved in the causation of thrombosis. E.F.A.s (essential fatty acids) play a fundamental role in keeping cell membranes fluid and flexible.

Single herbs: Cayenne, Comfrey, Evening Primrose Oil, Fish Oil, Garlic, Golden Seal, and Rose Hips.

Vitamins: B complex, C, E, Niacin, Inositol, and Choline.

Minerals: Calcium, Magnesium, and Selenium.

Also: (E.F.A.s) — Fish oils and cold pressed vegetable oils.

Helpful foods: Fish and fish liver oils, vegetable oils, oat bran, high fiber fruits, kelp, green tea, yogurt, and legumes.

Juices: Alfalfa, beet, blackberry, grape, parsley, and pineapple juice.

THRUSH

SPECIFICS: Thrush is a yeast-like fungus that inhabits the oral cavity. White sores form on the tongue, gums, and inside the cheeks. Diabetics are at great risk of contracting the fungus, so if a person is diagnosed with yeast infection, he or she should be checked for diabetes.

(Beneficial Remedies, Treatments, and Nutrients)

HERBAL COMBINATION: (Cantrol).

PHYSIOLOGIC ACTION: An excellent, well-balanced, formula of herbs and supplements which balance the system while killing yeast. It includes caprylic acid and anti-oxidants for the control and eventual elimination of the yeast infection.

Single herbs: Black Walnut, Caprinex, Garlicin, and Pau d'Arco.

Vitamins: Biotin and B complex.

Also: Caprilic Acid, Coenzyme Q10, L-Cysteine, Primadophilus, Primrose oil, and Salmon oil.

Helpful foods: Egg yolk, apricot, citrus fruits, beef kidney, beef liver, and vegetable and fish oils.

THYROID DISORDERS

SPECIFICS: Most thyroid disorders occur when there is an over or underproduction of hormones by the thyroid gland, resulting in lowered cellular metabolism.

In most thyroid disorders, the brain cells are effected and intellectual capacity is impaired. Problems with the thyroid gland can be the cause of many recurring illnesses, infections, and chronic fatigue.

(Beneficial Remedies, Treatments, and Nutrients)

HERBAL COMBINATION: (T).

PHYSIOLOGIC ACTION: Rich in natural vitamins and minerals, this excellent formula helps revitalize and promote healing of the thyroid glands, thus restoring metabolism balance. Helps the body store up needed vitality and energy.

Single herbs: Black Walnut, Irish Moss, Kelp, Mullein, and Parsley.

Vitamins: B1, B5, C, D, E, and F.

Minerals: Chlorine, Iodine, Potassium, and Zinc.

Also: Thyroid glandular.

Helpful foods: All fruits(citrus and other), black molasses, butter, cheese, beef, tuna, sardines, fish liver oils, beets, broccoli, carrots, vegetable oils, green leafy vegetables, soybeans, and sunflower seeds.

Juices: Clam and celery juice.

TICK BITE
(refer to Lyme disease - page 104)

TMJ SYNDROME
(refer to Temporomandibular Joint Syndrome page 156)

TINNITUS

SPECIFICS: This ailment is characterized by a buzzing, hissing, or ringing in one or both ears. ringing in the ears. Tinnitus is most often caused by impaired blood flow to the brain from clogged arteries and poor circulation.

(Beneficial Remedies, Treatments, and Nutrients)

HERBAL COMBINATIONS: (H Formula) (Ginkgold).

PHYSIOLOGIC ACTION: Contains herbs which strengthen the heart and builds the vascular system. When taken with Cayenne, it improves circulation and pulse rate, giving a warming and calming sensation to the ears.

Single herbs: Cayenne, Black Cohosh, Bayberry, Butchers Broom, Ginkgo, and Yarrow

Vitamins: A, B complex, B3, B6, C, and E.

Minerals: Calcium, Magnesium, Manganese, and Potassium.

Also: Bio-Strath, Coenzyme Q10, and Lecithin.

Helpful foods: All vegetables and vegetable oils, apples, bananas, citrus fruits, beets, broccoli, carrots, oat bran, soya beans, and whole wheat.

TIREDNESS
(refer to Fatigue "General" - page 66)

TONSILITIS

SPECIFICS: Inflammation of the tonsils; the glands of lymph tissue located on either side of the entrance to the throat. The most effective prevention and treatment for tonsillitis is a proper diet, high in vitamins, minerals, and protein.

(Beneficial Remedies, Treatments, and Nutrients)

HERBAL COMBINATION: (IF) (IGL).

PHYSIOLOGIC ACTION: Effective formulas that help cleanse toxins, combat infections, and reduce infection. Especially effective for healing the lymphatic system.

Single herbs: Bayberry Root, Echina Guard, Echinacea, Ginger Root and Pau d'Arco.

Vitamins and Minerals: A complete, one a day multi complex.

Also: Canaid herbal drink.

Helpful foods: Beef, broccoli, fruit(citrus and other), nuts, soybeans, spinach, sweet potatoes, turnip greens, unpolished rice, and whole grains.

TOOTHACHE
(refer to "Teeth and Gums" Page 155)

TOXOCARIASIS

SPECIFICS: An infestation of humans, with the larvae of toxocara canis, a threadlike worm that lives in the intestines of dogs. Early signs include diarrhea, loss of appetite, and rectal itching. If not eliminated they will result in the loss of weight, colon disorders, and anemia.

(Beneficial Remedies, Treatments, and Nutrients)

HERBAL COMBINATIONS: (Para-X) (Para-VF).

PHYSIOLOGIC ACTION: Useful in destroying and eliminating parasites, such as worms. Also helps relieve many kinds of skin problems. The Para-VF is liquid and is useful for children and the elderly who cannot swallow capsules.

WARNING: Do not use during pregnancy!

Single herbs: Black Walnut, Garlic, Pumpkin Seeds, Sage, Swedish Bitters, and Wormwood.

Vitamins: Folic Acid.

Minerals: A multi-mineral complex.

CHILDREN: Chamomile tea or raisins soaked in Senna tea for older children may be helpful.

TREMORS and TWITCHES

SPECIFICS: The most common cause of tremors and twitches is a deficiency of potassium, magnesium, and B vitamins. These nutrients are essential for the nerve impulses that pass to a muscle and control its movement.

(Beneficial Remedies, Treatments, and Nutrients)

Vitamins: B6, B12, Niacin, and B complex.

Minerals: Magnesium and Potassium.

Helpful foods: All vegetables, brewers yeast, apples, bananas, dates, figs, fish, liver, kidney, oat bran, wheat germ, and whole wheat products.

TRENCH MOUTH
(refer to Gingivitis - page 72)

TUBERCULOSIS (TB)

SPECIFICS: A highly contagious disease caused by the bacteria, Mycobacterium Tuberculosis.

It usually affects the lungs, but it may also involve other organs and tissues. The risk of contracting TB increases with an impaired immune system, an unbalanced diet, and close contact with someone infected. A diet high in protein and the essential vitamins and minerals will help prevent tuberculosis from recurring.

(Beneficial Remedies, Treatments, and Nutrients)

Single herbs: Echinacea and Pau d'Arco.

Vitamins: A, B complex, B2, B6, Folic acid, Pantothenic acid, C, D, and E.

Minerals: Zinc.

Also: L-Cysteine, L-Methionine, Germanium, and Protein.

Helpful foods: Apples, bananas, lean beef, black molasses, tuna, fish liver oils, cheese, non citrus fruit, mushrooms, and sweet potatoes.

TUMORS

SPECIFICS: Benign tumors are an abnormal growth of tissues that can occur anywhere in the body. These tumors do not spread and generally do not return after being removed. For information on malignant tumors, refer to "cancer" in this manual.

(Beneficial Remedies, Treatments, and Nutrients)

Single herbs: Dandelion, Kelp, Pau d'Arco, and Red Clover.

Vitamins: A, B5, B6, B complex, C, and E.

Minerals: A high potency multi-mineral.

Also: Coenzyme Q10, Germanium, Lecithin, Proteolytic enzymes, and Sheep Sorrel is an excellent poultice for external tumors.

Helpful foods: Aloe Vera, apples, bananas, broccoli, bran, carrots, citrus fruits, green leafy vegetables, soybeans, sweet potatoes, turnip greens, vegetable oils, lean red meat, and fish liver oils.

ULCERATIVE COLITIS

SPECIFICS: Ulcerative Colitis is often associated with, and made worse by psychological stress. Emotional upset should be avoided. Various herbs with multiple properties must be used to address the complexity of this situation.

Note: Avoid citrus juices. Bananas are very soothing and healing in ulcerative colitis. Primadophilus is effective in stabilizing flora in lower bowel.

(Beneficial Remedies, Treatments, and Nutrients)

Single herbs: Alfalfa, Bayberry, Chamomile, Caraway, Garlic, Reshi Mushroom, Plantain, Valerian, Wild Yam, and Yucca.

Vitamins: A, B6, Folic acid, Pantothenic acid, B complex, C, and E.

Minerals: Calcium, Iron, Magnesium, and Potassium.

Also: Multi-digestive and Proteolytic enzymes, Raw thymus glandular, and unsaturated fatty acids.

Helpful foods: Apples, bananas, lean beef, black molasses, tuna, fish liver oils, cheese, non citrus fruit, mushrooms, and sweet potatoes.

ULCERS (SKIN)

SPECIFICS: Skin ulcers are open sores on the skin that are generally caused as result of inadequate blood supply. Skin ulcers can be deep or shallow and are nearly always inflamed and painful.

(Beneficial Remedies, Treatments, and Nutrients)

HERBAL COMBINATION: (Myrrh – Golden seal).

PHYSIOLOGIC ACTION: Ingredients needed by the body to heal ulcers, cuts, wounds, bruises, sprains, and burns. Also good as a poultice for external wounds.

Vitamins: Folic acid, Pantothenic acid, C, and E.

Minerals: Multi-mineral complex.

Also: Aloe Vera and Unsaturated fatty acids.

Skin ulcers that do not heal — Vitamin E, topical application of comfrey root and/or tea leaf. Dress with a paste made of raw garlic on gauze for 8-10 hours. Take Vitamin A, C, Zinc and Calcium orally.

Helpful foods: Beef, fruits, nuts, unpolished rice, soybeans, spinach, vegetable oils, liver, and whole wheat.

ULCERS (STOMACH)

SPECIFICS: Stomach ulcers occur along the gastrointestinal tract and result when, during stress, the stomach is unable to secrete sufficient mucus, to protect against the strong acid essential for digestion. Symptoms of an ulcer are choking sensations, lower back pain, and stomach pain. Most ulcers are aggravated by the level of anxiety of the individual before eating.

(Beneficial Remedies, Treatments, and Nutrients)

HERBAL COMBINATION: (Myrrh – Gold Seal Plus).

Single herbs: Cayenne (stomach ulcers only), Golden Seal, Myrrh, Pau d'Arco, Red Raspberry, Slippery Elm Bark, Valerian, and White Oak Bark.

Vitamins: A, B complex, B2, B5, B6, B12, C, D, E, P, Choline, and Folic acid.

Minerals: Calcium, Manganese, and Zinc,

Also: Acidophilus, Chlorophyll, Raw Cabbage, Goat's milk, Brewer's yeast, and Halibut oil.

Refer to "Digestive Disorders" in this manual.

Helpful foods: Avocados, bananas, green leafy vegetables, red meat, bacon, chicken, cheese, fish liver oils, vegetable oils, oat bran, and whole grains.

Juices: Aloe Vera, celery, grapefruit, potato, and spinach juice.

UNDERWEIGHT

SPECIFICS: Treating undernourished people requires, first, stimulating the appetite. Consideration should be given to the eating environment, as well as the appearance and smell of food. People who have increased nutrient requirements would include victims of anorexia, burns, cancer treatments, hepatitis, and trauma.

(Beneficial Remedies, Treatments, and Nutrients)

Single herbs: Catnip, Fenugreek, Ginger root, Ginseng, Gota Kola, Saw Palmetto berries, Yucca, and bitter herbs such as those found in Swedish Bitters will stimulate appetite.

Vitamins: Multi-vitamins plus A and B complex.

Minerals: Multi-minerals plus Calcium, Copper, Magnesium, and Zinc.

Also: Brewers yeast, Bio-Strath, Digestive enzymes, Protein, and Unsaturated fatty acids.

Helpful foods: All dairy products, brewers yeast, beef, chicken, beer, fish and vegetable oils, potatoes, whole grain products, and nuts.

<u>URINARY TRACT</u> *(Infections)*

SPECIFICS: There are many problems that may occur in the urinary tract, however most of the problems are caused by infection. The symptoms of urinary tract infections are loss of appetite, chills, fever, frequency of urination, back pain, nausea, and vomiting.

(Beneficial Remedies, Treatments, and Nutrients)

HERBAL COMBINATION: (KB).

PHYSIOLOGIC ACTION: Extremely valuable in healing and strengthening the kidneys, bladder, and genito-urinary area. Useful to stop bed-wetting, but is a diuretic when congestion of the kidneys is indicated. Helps remove bladder, uterine, and urethral toxins.

WARNING: Intended for occasional use only. May cause green-yellow discoloration of urine.

Single herbs: Alfalfa, Barberry root, Catnip, Dandelion, Fennel, Ginger root, Goldenrod, Horsetail, Uva Ursi, and Wild Yam.

Vitamins: A, B complex, C, D, E, and Choline.

Minerals: Calcium, Magnesium, and Potassium.

Also: Digestive enzymes, Lecithin, L-Arginine, L-Methionine, Propolis, Uratonic, Watermelon, 3-way herb teas, and other Diuretic tablets.

Helpful foods: All vegetables, apples, bananas, broccoli, carrots, cheese and other dairy products, tuna, and fish liver oils, red meat, and sprouted seeds.

Juices: Asparagus, black currant, cranberry, celery, juniper berry, parsley, and pomegranate juice.

<u>URTICARIA</u>

SPECIFICS: This ailment is caused when the sap of the poison ivy or nettles touches the skin, it can cause persistent itching, rash, swelling, and blistering in sensitive people. The following nutrients will help alleviate the symptoms.

(Beneficial Remedies, Treatments, and Nutrients)

Single herbs: Echinacea, Goldenseal, and Lobelia.

Vitamins: A, C, and E.

Minerals: Zinc.

Helpful foods: Broccoli, carrots, citrus fruits, melon, fish liver oils, and vegetable oils.

VAGINAL PROBLEMS
(GYNECOLOGICAL PROBLEMS)

(Beneficial Remedies, Treatments, and Nutrients)

HERBAL COMBINATION: (Fem-Mend).

PHYSIOLOGIC ACTION: Menstrual regulator, tonic for genito-urinary system. Helpful for severe menstrual discomforts. Acts as an aid in rebuilding a malfunctioning reproductive system (Uterus, ovaries, fallopian tubes, etc.).

Single herbs: Aloe Vera, Blessed Thistle, Comfrey Root, Garlic, Ginger, Golden Seal Root, Red Raspberry, Slippery Elm Bark, Uva Ursi, and Yellow Dock Root.

Vitamins: A, B complex, C, and E.

Minerals: A complete multi-mineral complex.

Helpful foods: Dulse, pineapples, citrus fruits, broccoli, soybeans, spinach, sweet potatoes, turnip greens, vegetable oils, nuts, unpolished rice, and whole wheat.

VAGINITIS

SPECIFICS: An inflammation of the vagina, causing a white or yellow vaginal discharge, and a burning or itching sensation. The most common causes of vaginitis is diabetes, taking antibiotics, oral contraceptives, pregnancy, vitamin B deficiency, or a yeast infection.

(Beneficial Remedies, Treatments, and Nutrients)

Single herbs: Garlic, and Pau d'Arco.

HOMEOPATHIC COMBINATION: Vaginitis Formula.

Vitamins: A, B complex, B6, C, and D.

Minerals: Calcium and Magnesium.

Also: Acidophilus, Protein, and Unsaturated fatty acids.

Helpful foods: Egg yolk, apricot, citrus fruits, beef kidney, beef liver, and vegetable and fish liver oils.

VARICELLA
(refer to Chicken Pox - page 41)

VARICOSE VEINS

SPECIFICS: Age, lack of exercise, and chronic constipation are contributing factors to varicose veins. B and C vitamins are necessary for the maintenance of strong blood vessels. Research has indicated vitamin E improves circulation by dilating blood vessels.

(Beneficial Remedies, Treatments, and Nutrients)

Single herbs: Butchers Broom, Collinsonia, Hawthorn, Parsley, Horse chestnut, Marigold, Mistletoe, Witch Hazel, White Oak Bark, Uva Ursi, and Yarrow.

Vitamins: Multi-vitamin, plus B6, B12, B complex, C, and E.

Minerals: Potassium and Zinc.

Also: Brewer's yeast, Lecithin, Protein, and Unsaturated fatty acids.

Helpful foods: Apples, lean beef, broccoli, fruits(citrus and other),sprouted seeds, sunflower seeds, sweet potatoes, sardines, tuna, turnip greens, and yellow corn.

VENEREAL DISEASE

SPECIFICS: Gonorrhea is transmitted through sexual intimacy or from the mother to the newborn infant as it passes through the infected birth canal. Complications of gonorrhea may result in sterility in both sexes. Penicillin or another antibiotic is the usual treatment. In addition to medical treatment, an afflicted person should maintain a high nutrient diet to help repair the tissue damage that has occurred.

(Beneficial Remedies, Treatments, and Nutrients)

Single herbs: Echinacea, Goldenseal, Pau d'Arco and Suma.

Vitamins: B complex and K.

Minerals: Zinc.

Also: Acidophilus, Coenzyme Q10, Germanium, and Protein.

Helpful foods: All red meats, fruits, aloe vera, kelp, herring, oysters, liver, nuts, and yogurt.

VERTIGO

SPECIFICS: Vertigo occurs when the central nervous system receives conflicting messages from the inner ear, causing a sensation of lightheadedness or dizziness. The main causes are allergies, anemia, high or low blood pressure, lack of oxygen to the brain, stress, and nutritional deficiencies.

(Beneficial Remedies, Treatments, and Nutrients)

HERBAL COMBINATIONS: (ImmunAid) (B&B Extract) and (EchinaGuard).

PHYSIOLOGIC ACTION: Vertigo is generally caused by infections to the inner ear. ImmunAid boosts immunity, thereby helping with ear infections. EchinaGuard is a liquid. Echinacea extract is excellent for small children with ear infections. B&B Extract can be placed in the ear or taken internally and is used to aid poor equilibrium and nervous conditions.

Single herbs: Blue Cohosh, Echinacea, Garlic Oil, Garlic, Mullein Oil, Mullein, Skullcap, and St. Johns Wort.

Vitamins: A, B3, B6, B12, B complex, C, and E.

Minerals: Calcium and Magnesium.

Also: Canaid herbal drink, Coenzyme Q10, Germanium, Lecithin, Propolis, and Primadophilus.

Helpful foods: Lean red meat, carrots, green vegetables, citrus fruits, fish liver oils, herring, oysters, sardines, nuts, sprouted seeds, and sunflower seeds.

Note: When combating ear infections, it is imperative to exclude allergen foods from the diet. This is particularly true of all dairy products.

VINCENT'S DISEASE
(refer to Gingivitis - page 72)

VIRAL INFECTIONS

SPECIFICS: Viruses are smaller than bacteria and live on the body's cell enzymes. Most viral infections cause chills, fever, headache, and muscular aches and pains.

(Beneficial Remedies, Treatments, and Nutrients)

Single herbs: Catnip, Echinacea, Garlic, Kelp, and Pau d'Arco.

Vitamins: A, B complex, B5, and C.

Minerals: A high potency multi-mineral plus Zinc.

Also: Germanium, L-Cysteine, Proteolytic enzymes, Canaid herbal drink, and Raw thymus.

Helpful foods: Apricots, bananas, citrus fruits, broccoli, carrots, celery, corn, green leafy vegetables, bacon, beef, chicken, and fish liver oils.

Juices: Celery, grapefruit, lemon, and parsley juice.

VITILIGO

SPECIFICS: A skin condition characterized by white patches surrounded by a dark border. Often thyroid malfunction is behind this disorder.

(Beneficial Remedies, Treatments, and Nutrients)

HERBAL COMBINATION: (T).

PHYSIOLOGIC ACTION: Rich in natural vitamins and minerals, this excellent formula helps revitalize and promote healing of the thyroid glands, thus restoring metabolism balance. Helps the body store up needed vitality and energy.

Single herbs: Black Walnut, Irish Moss, Kelp, Mullein, and Parsley.

Vitamins: B1, B5, C, D, E, and F.

Minerals: Chlorine, Iodine, Potassium, and Zinc.

Also: Thyroid glandular, and Essential fatty acids.

Helpful foods: All fruits(citrus and other), black molasses, butter, cheese, beef, tuna, sardines, fish liver oils, beets, broccoli, carrots, vegetable oils, green leafy vegetables, soybeans, and sunflower seeds.

Juices: Clam and celery juice.

WARTS *(Common)*

SPECIFICS: Warts are highly contagious, rough, irregular skin growths. They can be spread by trimming, picking, touching, or shaving. Typically they do not cause pain or itching. Proper nutrition and the supplements listed below will control or eliminate common warts.

(Beneficial Remedies, Treatments, and Nutrients)

Single herbs: Echinacea, Garlic, Golden Seal, and Pau d' Arco.

Vitamins: A, B complex, C, and E.

Minerals: Zinc.

Also: L-Cysteine, and 28000 IU vitamin E oil applied twice a day is an effective treatment.

Helpful foods: Fish and fish liver oils, all vegetables and vegetable oils, mushrooms, unpolished rice, fruit, and whole wheat.

WATER RETENTION

SPECIFICS: Disorders that cause water retention are sodium retention, congestive heart failure, weak kidneys, varicose veins, and protein and thiamine deficiencies.

(Beneficial Remedies, Treatments, and Nutrients)

HERBAL COMBINATION: (KB).

PHYSIOLOGIC ACTION: KB acts as a mild diuretic to rid the body of excessive water.

Single herbs: Buchu, Cranberry, Dandelion, Juniper, Parsley, and Uva Ursi.

Vitamins: B6 and C.

Minerals: Calcium and Potassium.

Also: Limited consumption of common table salt.

Helpful foods: Bananas, citrus fruits, cheese, nuts, oat bran, sweet potatoes, and turnip greens.

WEIGHT CONTROL *(Overweight)*

SPECIFICS: A person who has twenty percent excess body fat over the norm for their age, build, and height is considered overweight. Losing weight is a matter of consciously regulating the types and amount of food eaten and increasing daily activity.

(Beneficial Remedies, Treatments, and Nutrients)

HERBAL COMBINATIONS: (SKC) or (Herbal Slim).

PHYSIOLOGIC ACTION: A special, well-balanced, combination that helps control your appetite, dissolve excess fat, ease stress and anxiety, gently cleanse the bowels, eliminate excess water, and in conjunction with your diet and exercise program, helps you lose weight naturally. Safe and effective.

Single herbs: Guar Gum, Konjac Root, and Yucca.

Vitamins: A, C, and E.

Minerals: A complete multi-mineral complex.

Also: Super D's tea, Slim tea, Spirulina diet, Bee Pollen, and Grapefruit Plus.

Helpful foods: Citrus fruits, melon, fish liver oils, green leafy vegetables, and oat bran.

WEIGHT GAIN

SPECIFICS: Treating undernourished people requires, first, stimulating the appetite. Consideration should be given to the eating environment, as well as the appearance and smell of food. People who have increased nutrient requirements would include victims of anorexia, burns, cancer treatments, hepatitis, and trauma.

(Beneficial Remedies, Treatments, and Nutrients)

Single herbs: Catnip, Fenugreek, Ginger root, Ginseng, Gota Kola, Saw Palmetto berries, and bitter herbs such as those found in Swedish Bitters will stimulate appetite.

Vitamins: Multi-vitamins plus A and B complex.

Minerals: Multi-minerals plus Calcium, Copper, Magnesium, and Zinc.

Also: Brewers yeast, Bio-Strath, Digestive enzymes, Protein, and Unsaturated fatty acids.

Helpful foods: All dairy products, brewers yeast, beef, chicken, beer, fish and vegetable oils, potatoes, whole grain products, and nuts.

WHOOPING COUGH

SPECIFICS: A distressing infectious disease, also known as pertussis which mainly affects young children and infants. The main features of the illness are paroxysms of coughing often ending in a characteristic "whoop".

(Beneficial Remedies, Treatments, and Nutrients)

HERBAL COMBINATION: (A-P).

PHYSIOLOGIC ACTION: A natural way to ease chronic pain associated with nervous tension, spasms, and whooping cough.

Single herbs: Elecampane, Horehound, Kalmin, Mouse Ear, Sundew, Valerian Root, Wild Cherry Bark, and Wild Lettuce.

Vitamins: Multi-vitamin complex.

Minerals: Multi-mineral complex plus Zinc.

Helpful foods: Apples, citrus fruit, celery, herring, oysters, and turnip greens.

Juices: Apple, celery, and watercress.

WORMS

SPECIFICS: Worms live in the gastrointestinal tract. Early signs include diarrhea, loss of appetite, and rectal itching.
If not eliminated they will result in the loss of weight, colon disorders, and anemia. Causes include ingestion of eggs or larvae from partially cooked meat, improper disposal of human waste, and walking barefoot on contaminated soil.

(Beneficial Remedies, Treatments, and Nutrients)

HERBAL COMBINATIONS: (Para-X) (Para-VF).

PHYSIOLOGIC ACTION: Useful in destroying and eliminating parasites, such as worms. Also helps relieve many kinds of skin problems. The Para-VF is liquid and is useful for children and the elderly who cannot swallow capsules.

WARNING: Do not use during pregnancy!

Single herbs: Black Walnut, Garlic, Pumpkin Seeds, Sage, Swedish Bitters, and Wormwood.

Vitamins: Folic Acid.

Minerals: A multi-mineral complex.

CHILDREN: Chamomile tea or raisins soaked in Senna tea for older children may be helpful.

Helpful foods: Asparagus, brewers yeast, broccoli, lettuce, lima beans, liver, mushrooms, nuts, and spinach.

WRINKLES
(refer to Skin Problems - page 149)

YEAST INFECTION

SPECIFICS: A fungus such as candida albicans inhabits the genital tract, intestines, mouth and throat. Yeast infections affect both men and women; when the fungus infects the vagina it results in vaginitis; when it infects the oral cavity, it is called thrush. Diabetics are at great risk of contracting the fungus, so if a person is diagnosed with yeast infection, he or she should be checked for diabetes.

(Beneficial Remedies, Treatments, and Nutrients)

HERBAL COMBINATIONS: (Garlicin) (Control, Caprinex).

PHYSIOLOGIC ACTION: Excellent well-balanced formulas for control and eventual elimination of candida overgrowth.

Single herbs: Black Walnut, Garlic, and Pau d'Arco.
Vitamins: A, C, E, and Biotin.
Minerals: Calcium and Magnesium.
Also: Primrose oil, Protein, and Primadophilus.

HERBAL DOSAGES

You should only use the dosages recommended by the manufacturer as the strengths can vary. The quantities and frequencies written on the labels are for adults weighing approximately 150 lbs. When using herbal remedies for children or the elderly, the use should be decreased. Herbal capsules may be prepared as a tea. To make sure that the herbs are properly assimilated, they should be taken with a full glass of water.

VITAMINS & MINERALS

Continual debate rages over what is an (adequate) daily intake of vitamins and minerals. The guide below is just that — a guide only. RDA and Margin of Allowances, are based on the minimum needs of an average adult 23 to 50 years of age, with no special health problems.

VITAMINS		*RDA for adult, 23-50 **	*Margin of Allowance***
Vitamin A	Adults	4,000 IU	5-10 times RDA **
	Children	2,000 IU	4,000 IU
	Infants	1,400 IU	2,000 IU
Beta-carotene	Adults	7,500 IU	5-10 times RDA ***
B complex	See individual B vitamins - Relatively non-toxic		
(B1)	Men	1.4 mg	200 times RDA **
Thiamin	Women	1.0 mg	200 times RDA **
	Children	.7 to 1.2 mg	n/a
	Infants	.3 to .5 mg	n/a
(B2)	Men	1.6 mg	588 times RDA **
Riboflavin	Women	1.2 mg	588 times RDA **
	Children	.8 to 1.4 mg	n/a
	Infants	.4 to .6 mg	n/a
(B3)	Men	16 mg	50 times RDA **
Niacin	Women	13 mg	50 times RDA **
	Children	9 mg	n/a
	Infants	6 mg	n/a

Dosages

VITAMINS		RDA for adult, 23-50 *	Margin of Allowance**
(B5)	Adults	10 mg	100 times RDA **
Pantothenic	Children	3 to 7 mg	n/a
acid	Infants	2 to 3 mg	n/a
(B6)	Men	2.2 mg	900 times RDA **
Pyridoxine	Women	2 mg	900 times RDA **
	Children	.9 to 1.8 mg	n/a
	Infants	.3 to .6 mg	n/a
(B9)	Adults	180 to 200 mcg	1000 times RDA **
Folic acid	Children	100 mcg	n/a
	Infants	10 to 40 mcg	n/a
(B12)	Adults	6 mcg	25 to 100 mg ****
Cobalamin			
(B13)		Not available in the U.S.A.	
Orotic acid		Available as calcium orotate outside of the U.S.A.	
(B15)	Adults	50 mg ***	100 mg ****
Calc. Pangamate			
(B17)	Adults	.25 g ***	1g ****
Laetrile			
Choline	Adults	900 mg ***	1 to 5g ****
Inositol	Adults	250 mg ***	500-1000 mg ****
PABA	Adults	100 mg ***	1000 mg ****
Para-amino benzoic Acid			
Vitamin C	Adults	60 mg	33-83 times RDA **
	Children	45 to 50 mg	n/a
	Infants	35 mg	n/a

VITAMINS		RDA for adult, 23-50 *	Margin of Allowance**	
Vitamin D	Adults	400 IU	2.5 to 5 times RDA	**
	Children	400 IU	2.5 times RDA	***
	Infants	200 IU	2.5 times RDA	***
Vitamin E	Men	15 IU	40 times RDA	**
	Women	12 IU	40 times RDA	**
	Children	7 to 12 IU	20 times RDA	***
	Infants	4 to 6 IU	15 times RDA	***
Vitamin F Unsaturated fatty acids	Adults	100 mg	1,000 mg	***
Vitamin H Biotin	Adults	250 mcg	1,000 mcg	***
	Children	100 mcg	200 mcg	***
	Infants	35 to 50 mcg	n/a	
Vitamin K - 1	Adults	65 to 80 mcg	10 to 15 times RDA	***
Vitamin K - 2	Children	20 to 50 mcg	5 to 10 times RDA	***
	Infants	10 to 20 mcg	3 to 5 times RDA	***
Vitamin K - 3 Menadione	Adults	65-80 mcg	500 mcg	***
Vitamin P Bioflavonoids	Adults	12 mg	33-83 times RDA	**
Vitamin T Sesame seeds		n/a	n/a	
Vitamin U Raw cabbage		n/a	n/a	

DOSAGES

MINERALS		RDA for adult, 23-50 *		Margin of Allowance**	
Boron	Adults	2 mg		3 to 6 mg	***--
Calcium	Adults	800 mg		10 times RDA	**
	Children	800 to 1200 mg		10 times RDA	**
	Infants	360 to 540 mg		n/a	
Chlorine	Adults	500 mg		1500 mg	****
Chromium	Adults	.05 to .2 mg	***	.2 to .6 mg	***
	Children	.02 to .2 mg	***	n/a	
	Infants	.01 to .06 mg	***	n/a	
Cobalt	Adults	5 to 8 mcg	***	n/a	
Copper	Adults	2 to 3 mg		5.5 times RDA	**
	Children	1 to 3 mg		n/a	
	Infants	.5 to 1 mg		n/a	
Fluorine	Adults	1.5 mg	***	4 mg	****
	Children	.5 mg	***	2.5 mg	****
	Infants	.1 mg	***	1 mg	****
Iodine	Adults	150 mcg		1000 mcg	***
	Children	70 to 150 mcg		300 mcg	***
	Infants	40 to 50 mcg		100 mcg	***
Iron	Men	10 mg		5.5 times RDA	**
	Women	18 mg		5.5 times RDA	**
	Children	15 to 18 mg		n/a	
	Infants	10 to 15 mg		n/a	

MINERALS		RDA for adult, 23-50 *	Margin of Allowance**
Lithium		n/a	n/a
Magnesium	Men	350 mg	15 times RDA **
	Women	300 mg	15 times RDA **
	Children	150 to 300 mg	5 times RDA ***
	Infants	50 to 70 mg	n/a
Manganese	Adults	2.5 to 5 mg	15 to 30 mg ****
	Children	1 to 5 mg	n/a
	Infants	.5 to 1 mg	n/a
Molybdenum	Adults	.15 to .25 mg ***	.5 mg ****
	Children	.05 to .25 mg ***	.5 mg ****
	Infants	.03 to .05 mg ***	.08 mg ****
Nickel		n/a	Excessive intake may be toxic.
Phosphorus	Adults	1000 mg	10 times RDA **
	Children	800 to 1200 mg	5 times RDA ***
	Infants	240 to 360 mg	n/a
Potassium	Adults	1875 to 5625 mg	No known toxicity.
	Children	550 to 4575 mg	n/a
	Infants	350 to 1275 mg	n/a
Selenium	Men	.07 mg	.2 mg ***
	Women	.05 mg	.15 mg ***
	Children	.02 mg	.1 mg ***
	Infants	.01 mg	.06 mg ***
Silicon	Adults	n/a	No side effects have been found to date.

Dosages

MINERALS		RDA for adult, 23-50 *		Margin of Allowance**	
Sodium	Adults	1100 to 3300 mg		8 grams	****
	Children	325 to 2700 mg		2 to 6 grams	****
	Infants	115 to 750 mg		1 to 2 grams	****
Sulfur	Adults		n/a	Inorganic sulfur can be toxic.	
Vanadium form.	Adults		n/a	Can be toxic in synthetic	
Zinc	Adults	15 mg		33 times RDA	**
	Children	10 to 15 mg		15 times RDA	***
	Infants	3 to 5 mg		5 times RDA	***

*   U.S.A. (Recommended Daily Allowances) are based on estimates by the National Academy of Sciences and National Research Council.

**   Adapted from John Hathcock's "Quantitative Evaluation of Vitamin Safety," Pharmacy Times, May 1985.

***   Estimate only — from Global Health Research on data available.

****   Usual therapeutic dose.

RDAs and Margin of Allowances courtesy of the
"Natural Life Magazine" Burnaby, B.C., Canada.

BIBLIOGRAPHY

Adams, Ruth. - *Vitamin E, Wonder Worker of the 70's.* New York, U.S.A: Larchmont books 1972.

Adams, Ruth. - *Body, Mind, & B Vitamins.* New York, U.S.A: Larchmont books 1972.

Airola, Paavo. - *Are You Confused?* Ariz. U.S.A: Health Plus, 1974.

Airola, Paavo. - *Cancer Causes, Prevention and Treatments.* Ariz. U.S.A: Health Plus, 1972.

Airola, Paavo. - *How to Get Well.* Ariz. U.S.A: Health Plus, 1974.

Alexeev, U.E. - *Herbal Plants of the U.S.S.R.* Moscow, U.S.S.R: MISL, 1971.

Allshorn, George, E. - *Domestic Homeopathic Practice.* London, England: Houston and Write, 1871.

Ancowitz, Aurthur. - *Strokes and Their Prevention.* New York, U.S.A: Jove Publications, 1982.

Andrews, Ralph W. - *Indian Primitive.* New York, U.S.A: Bonanza Books, 1962.

Atkins, Robert C. - *Dr. Atkins' Nutrition Breakthrough.* New York, U.S.A: Bantom Books 1981.

Bakuleff, A. N. and Petroff, F.N. *Popular Medical Encyclopedia.* Moscow, U.S.A: Bolshaya Soviet Encyclopedia, 1965.

Bailey, Herbert. - *Vitamin E: Your Key to a Healthy Heart.* New York, U.S.A: Ark Books, 1970.

Barker, Eillis J. - *New Lives for Old.* London, England: Homeopathic Publishing Co. Ltd., 1949.

Basu, T.K. - *About Mothers, Children and Their Nutrition.* London, England: Thorsons Publishing, 1981.

Bender, George, A. - *Great Moments in Medicine.* Michigan, U.S.A: Park Davis, 1961.

Benjamin, Harry. - *Unorthodox Healing Versus Medical Science.* London, England: Health for All Publishing Co., 1951.

Bodman, Frank. - *Insights into Homeotherapeutics.* London, England: Beakonsfield Publisher, 1990.

Bogorad, B.B. - *Dictionary of Biological Terms.* Moscow, U.S.S.R. Ministry of Education, 1963.

Borsaak, Henry. - *Vitamins:* What they are and How They Can Effect You. New York, U.S.A: Pyramid Books, 1971.

Brennan, R.O. - *Nutrigenetics.* New York, U.S.A: New American Library, 1977.

Brewster, Dorothy Patricia. - *You Can Breastfeed Your Baby.* PA U.S.A: Rodale Press, 1979.

Bibliography

Davis, Adelle. - *Let's Get Well.* New York, U.S.A: New American Library, 1972.

Davis, Adelle. and Marshall Mandell. - *Let's Have Healthy Children.* New York, U.S.A: New American Library, 1979.

Dastur, J.F. - *Medicinal Plants of India and Pakistan.* Bombay, India: Taraporevala Sons and Co., 1962.

De-Vries, Arnold. - *Primitive Man and His Food.* Chicago, U.S.A: Chandler Book Co., 1952.

Dewey, W.A. - *Practical Homeopathic Therapeutics.* New Delhi, India: Jain Publishing Co., No Date.

Doole, Louise E. - *Herbs and Garden Ideas.* New York, U.S.A: Sterling Publishing Co., 1964.

Dunne, Lavon J. - *Nutrition Almanac.* New York, U.S.A: McGraw-Hill Book Co., 1979.

Ebon, Martin. - *The Truth About Vitamin E.* New York, U.S.A: Bantam Books, 1972.

Ehrlich, David, and George Wolf. - *The Bowel Book.* New York, U.S.A: Schocken Books, 1981.

Farrandez, V. L. - *Guia de Medicina Vegetal.* Celoni, Spain: J. Impentor, 1967.

Farrington, E.A. - *Clinical Materia Medica.* New Delhi, India: Jain Publishers, 1981.

Feingold, Ben W. - *Why Your Child is Hyperactive.* New York, U.S.A: Random House, 1975.

Fortisevn, Zeke. - *Global Herb Manual.* Alberta, Canada: Global Health Ltd., 1992.

Graham, Judy. - *Multiple Sclerosis.* Wellingborough, England: Thorsons Publishers, 1982.

Grey, Madeline. - *The Changing Years.* New York, U.S.A: Doubleday, 1981.

Hutchens, Alma R. - *Indian Herbalogy of North America.* Michigan, U.S.A: Ann Arbor, 1982

Jensen, Bernard. - *Seeds and Sprouts for Life.* California, U.S.A: Jenson's Nutrition and Health Prod., No date.

Jouanny, Jacques. - *The Essentials of Homeopathic Materia Medica.* Lyon, France: Laboratoires Boiron, 1984.

Kadans, Joseph M. - *Modern Encyclopedia of Herbs.* New York, U.S.A: Parker publishing Co. 1970.

Katz, Marcella. - *Vitamins, Food, and Your Health.* U.S.A: Public Affairs Committee, 1975.

Kushi, Michio. - *The Book of Macrobiotics.* Tokyo, Japan: Japan Publications, 1977.

Kushi, Michio. - *The Book of Oriental Diagnosis..* Tokyo, Japan: Japan Publications, 1980.

Lesser, Michael. - *Nutrition and Vitamin Therapy.* New York, U.S.A: Grove Press, 1980.

Locke, David M. - *Enzymes-The Agents of Life.* New York, U.S.A: Crown Press, 1971.

Martin, Marvin. - *Great Vitamin Mystery.* IL, U.S.A: National Dairy Council, 1978.

Mindell, Earl. - *Mindell's Vitamin Bible.* New York, U.S.A: Warner Books, 1980.

Mindell, Earl. - *Mindell's Herb Bible.* New York, U.S.A: Simon & Schuster, 1992.

Meyer, Joseph E. - *The Herbalist.* Illinois, U.S.A: Meyerbooks, 1991.

Newbold, H.L. - *Mega-Nutrients for Your Nerves.* New York, U.S.A: Berkley Publishing, 1981.

Nyholt, David H. - *The Athlete's Bible.* Alberta, Canada: Global Health Ltd., 1989.

Nyholt, David H. *The Complete Natural Health Encyclopedia.* Alberta, Canada: Global Health Ltd., 1994.

Nyholt, David H. - *The Vitamin & Herb Guide.* Alberta, Canada: Global Health Ltd., 1992.

Passwater, Ritchard A. - *Selenium as Food and Medicine.* Conn., U.S.A: Keats Publishing Co., 1980.

Pearson, Durk, and Sandy Shaw - *Life Extension.* New York, U.S.A: Warner Books, 1982.

Roberts, Frank. - *The Encyclopedia of Digestive Disorders.* London, England: Thorsons Publishers, No Date.

Rodale, J.I. - *Be a Healthy Mother, Have a Healthy Baby.* PA, U.S.A: Rodale Books, 1973.

Rodenberg, Harold. and Feldzaman, A.N. - *Doctors Book of Vitamin Therapy:* Megavitamins for Health. New York, U.S.A: Putnam's, 1974.

Sokol, Steve. - *The Fitness Formula.* Alberta, Canada: Global Health Ltd., 1992.

Taberner, P.V. - *Aphrodisiacs: The Science and the Myth.* PA, U.S.A: University of Pennsylvania, 1985.

Thomas, Clayton L. - *Taber's Cyclopedia Medical Dictionary* 12th ed. PA, U.S.A: Davis Co., 1973

Vogel, Virgil J. - *American Indian Medicine.* Oklahoma, U.S.A: University of Oklahoma, 1970.

Wade, Carlson. - *Helping Your Health with Enzymes.* New York, U.S.A: Universal-Award House, 1971.

Wheatly, Michael. - *About Nutrition.* London, England: Thorsons, 1971.

INDEX

400
COMMON AILMENTS

INDEX

INDEX

INDEX

INDEX

DOSAGES

GLOSSARY

BIBLIOGRAPHY

GLOBAL HEALTH BOOKS

NEW

Drugs and Beyond

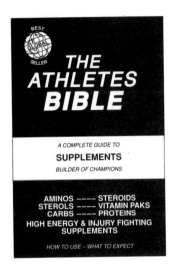

Drugs & Beyond

A family approach to abused and misused drugs.
by Global Health Research
$11.95 U.S.A. / $14.95 Cdn.

An informative and heavily researched book, construed in cooperation with some of the top drug specialists in the world, to help the general public fully understand the consequences of abused and misused drugs. This book contains illustrations and clearly designed charts to give you more information in less reading time. It covers the full spectrum of legal and illegal drugs from caffeine to heroin, the newest synthetic drugs, and the latest natural alternatives and scientific breakthroughs for the treatments of drug addictions.

The Athlete's Bible
The proper nutrition to boost your athletic abilities.
by David Nyholt
$9.95 U.S.A./ $11.95 Cdn.

If you are an Olympic, professional, or recreational athlete, this is the book for you. Concise, up to date information on high performance sport nutrition, aminos, steroids, sterols, vitamins, carbs, proteins, high energy, and injury fighting supplements. Enables you to boost your athletic abilities, promote safe muscle tissue growth, increase strength and stamina. Enhance energy levels through proper nutritional supplementation and reach your highest possible potential, without harmful drugs or chemical additives.

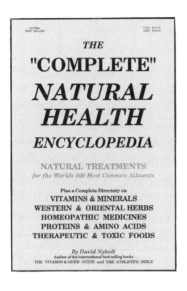

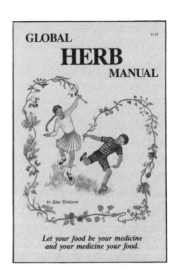

The "Complete" Natural Health Encyclopedia

A Natural Information Giant
by David Nyholt
$14.95 U.S.A./$18.95 Cdn.

This concise, comprehensive, and easy to use natural health encyclopedia, is designed to give you more practical information in less reading time. It features the latest breakthroughs in natural health science. Proven and effective natural treatments for over 350 common ailments. Over 300 western and oriental herbs with their up to date characteristics. 110 Homeopathic remedies. The healing and toxic qualities of 130 foods and spices. Clearly designed charts on Vitamins, Minerals, Amino Acids, Tissue Salts, and the recommended daily allowances. This book is a must for all people wishing to restore health and prevent premature aging.

Global Herb Manual

New Sixth Edition
The Latest in Herbal Science
by Zeke Fortisevn
$4.95 U.S.A./$5.95 Cdn.

This manual is a vast storehouse of knowledge on herbs. Discover the amazing healing and preventative properties of ancient and modern herbs. Plants are mankind's chief method of healing and main source of medicine. This simplified book contains all of the common herbs and characteristics, the effective herbal combinations, extracts, oils and syrups, and their specific functions. Proven herbal cleansing diets, over 50 herbal treatments for the world's most common ailments, plus a comprehensive index and a complete herbal glossary.

**Books are available directly from the publishers.
Send list price plus $2.50 for shipping and handling.**

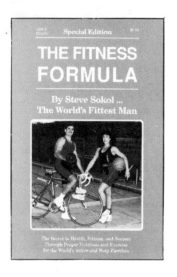

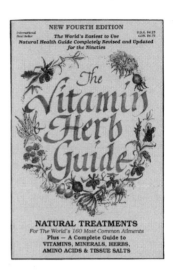

The Fitness Formula
A Must For The World's Active and Busy Families
by Steve Sokol
$4.95 U.S.A./ $5.95 Cdn.

The Secret to Health, Fitness, and Success. Steve Sokol is not only a talented writer and spokesman for numerous health related associations, but also holds over twenty world fitness records. In this book Steve shares with you his proven techniques designed for people of all skill levels, to increase energy levels, mental alertness, health, and fitness. A sensible plan to feel and look your personal best. Building confidence and success through proper nutrition and exercise.

The Vitamin & Herb Guide
Revised Fifth Edition
By David Nyholt
$4.95 U.S.A./ $5.95 Cdn.

This highly acclaimed International best seller is the most concise, and easiest to use natural health guide in the world today. Designed to give you more information in less reading time. The quick scan index allows you to find what you want and need to know instantly. features comprehensive quick reference charts on all vitamins, minerals, herbs, amino acids, tissue salts and effective natural treatments for 160 common ailments. That's precisely why busy people around the world rely on - - -
The Vitamin & Herb Guide.